The ACL Guidebook

A Patient's Point of View

By

Shai Simonson

Table of Contents

Acknowledgements

My surgeon, Dr. Eric Berkson, supported this project throughout with many emails and conversations, explaining a great deal of the medical information in this book in layperson's terms. He is not only a top-level surgeon, but also a thoughtful doctor with a refined bedside manner and a gift for teaching. More than five years after my surgery, I am deeply grateful for a knee that feels as good as it did before my injury.

I thank all the volunteers who permitted me to share their personal ACL stories. Thanks also to Astitva Srivastava for designing the book cover.

And, thanks to my wife, Andrea, for nursing me patiently back to health, tolerating my stubborn and aggressive approach to rehab, proofreading the entire book, and offering many helpful suggestions.

Disclaimer

The content of this book is not intended to be a substitute for professional medical advice, diagnosis, or treatment. Always seek the advice of your physician or other qualified health provider with any questions you may have regarding a medical condition.

Introduction

"I hope they find a cure, but if it involves months of intense physical therapy, I think I'll pass." Homer Simpson

Every year in the US, an estimated quarter of a million people, mostly athletes, tear their anterior cruciate ligaments (ACLs), and more than 150,000 undergo ACL replacement surgery. The injuries of famous athletes may make the evening news, but the vast majority of ACL injuries are suffered by the not-so-rich and famous: high school athletes, college athletes, weekend warriors, aspiring gymnasts, recreational soccer players and football players, basketball and baseball players, tennis buffs, rock climbers, dancers, volleyball players, and so on. Every individual's story of ACL injury is an ordeal to him or her, whether or not it affects the Super Bowl, the NBA championship, the Olympics, or the Masters. If you have torn your ACL and you want to know what's next, then this book is for you.

There are lots of online resources about torn ACLs. There are forums for sharing stories, posting questions, and reading/writing answers. There are sites focusing on the anatomy, on the surgery, and on the rehab. You can even watch a live surgery with running commentary on YouTube. When I tore my ACL, I visited many sites; I read and posted on the forums; I watched the surgery video; and I pestered doctors with dozens of questions. After months, I gathered enough information to decide how to treat my injury effectively. Partnering with my surgeon Dr. Eric Berkson, I wrote this book to inform, educate, entertain, and ultimately make it easier for other people to manage their ACL injuries.

This book explains everything you ever wanted to know about the human knee, the ACL, and ACL injuries and treatments. It is the guidebook I wish I had had when I tore my ACL. The more you know about your knee and your ACL, the better equipped you will be to make important decisions about whether or not to have surgery, and the more committed you will be to the necessary rehabilitation whether or not you choose to undergo surgery. After reading this book, you will know the answers to the following list of questions and many more.

- What is the ACL?
- What is its purpose, and what are the implications of a torn ACL?
- How and why does an ACL get torn?
- How do you know that you have a torn ACL?
- What are your options and treatments when you tear your ACL?
- How common is a partial tear of the ACL?
- Is there a difference in the treatment for a complete tear versus a partial tear?
- What are the expectations after surgery and rehabilitation?
- What are the risks of surgery and what are the risks of avoiding surgery?
- Can an ACL be surgically repaired or is replacement necessary?
- How does age affect options for treatment?
- Can you be active without an ACL?
- How long and hard is the rehab?
- How long will I be out of work?
- How bad is the pain from surgery and subsequent rehab?

The book is organized in a practical manner. Those who want quick access to the relevant information can consult the questions and answers in Chapter 4. For a more leisurely, personal, and amusing tour of ACL injuries, you can read through the story of my injury and subsequent rehabilitation. To get perspective, you can read stories of other people with ACL injuries and try to find one that most closely matches your own. If you are curious to learn more about the science of surgery, you can study the fascinating 100-year long history of ACL surgery and its outcomes. Finally, we hope you will be entertained throughout, so that at the very least, the book will serve as a pleasant distraction to the challenges that await you.

Chapter 1 – Famous ACLs

"I definitely don't wish that injury on my worst enemy. That was definitely a tough one."

Wes Welker, wide receiver New England Patriots and Denver Broncos

At the end of the 2009 NFL season, the New England Patriots were playing the Houston Texans in their last regular game of the season. Just six minutes into the first quarter, 3rd down and four, Tom Brady takes the snap on his own 42-yard line. Wide receiver Wes Welker runs an in-and-out option pattern, and Brady throws a short pass caught by Welker just past the line of scrimmage. Welker is a slot receiver and an expert on this kind of "catch and run" play. His ability to receive the ball, cut, and make quick moves is a big threat to opposing defenses. Not only can he turn a short pass into a big gain with extra running yards, but his ability to do this opens up longer routes for his teammate Randy Moss, especially with Tom Brady as quarterback.

Welker gets a block and heads five or six yards up an open field. He reaches the first down marker and continues past midfield to the Texans' 46-yard line where the 5' 9" 185 pound Welker is met by the Texans' 6' 2" 225-pound strong safety, Bernard Pollard. There is a lot of room to move, and it's one on one. Welker cuts sharply and presses his left leg hard into the ground. Just as it looks as if he is going to elude the would be tackler, Welker's left knee bends inward awkwardly, and he inexplicably falls to the ground, curls up in a ball, and grabs his knee in pain. Pollard, standing nearby, never even touched him. Welker is not getting up and the commentators start to speculate.

They wonder about the seriousness of the injury. In another week, the Patriots are headed to the playoffs against the Baltimore Ravens and they cannot afford to lose Welker for that game. Trainers rush in from the sidelines. Coach Bill Belichik, quarterback Tom Brady, and wide receiver Randy Moss are also crowding around Welker. Finally, Welker stands up on his own, grimacing, and walks off the field assisted by two trainers. He sits down and starts to cry while thousands of nervous fans in the stands and on TV watch, wonder, and listen to the commentators.

Kevin Harlan: "This guy is as important as any player on this team the way he has been catching, and running after the catches, and impacting the opposing defense."

Solomon Wilcots: "He's very emotional. I mean he's hurt. I've been in that situation. I've seen players that emotional. They know that there's something quite not right." [1]

Indeed, Welker isn't crying just because of the pain. He seems to understand what his trainers don't yet know – that he will not walk off this injury; that his season is over. His team, whose momentum was just starting to swell, will be going to the playoffs without him. With Welker out of the game, the Patriots lose to the Texans by a score of 34 to 27, and without Welker, a week later in the first round of the 2009 NFL playoffs, the Patriots lose 33 to 14 to the Baltimore Ravens.

Welker tore the ACL in his left knee. The anterior cruciate ligament (ACL) is one of four major ligaments that help stabilize the knee. Missing an ACL, an athlete cannot cut or pivot sharply without falling and further injuring other ligaments or tissue in the knee. There is no hope for regeneration of a completely torn ACL, and repairing an ACL is not a viable option. A *repaired* ACL often tears and fails again.

Twenty or thirty years ago, a torn ACL often marked the end of an athlete's career. He/she could swim, jog, or cycle, and likely handle any activity that requires simple forward and backward motion. However, participation in sports that demand rotations and/or quick side-to-

---

[1] NFL on CBS http://www.youtube.com/watch?v=-RK4qhQWIUo

side motions would be impossible. Cutting, jumping, pivoting, or rotating with a torn ACL can result in a knee "giving out," causing further injury and pain. A person with an untreated torn, stretched, injured, or weakened ACL is sometimes said to have a "trick knee," meaning that the knee will occasionally, and unpredictably, buckle under various strains and efforts.

The history of ACL repair and replacement is a hundred years old, and in that time many different options have been studied. Although ACL *repair* has proven unreliable, the outcomes today for surgical ACL *replacement* are excellent. And, although *artificial* replacements have *not* been effective, natural replacements have great outcomes. Popular natural options today for ACL replacement include an athlete's patellar tendon or hamstring tendon, and various cadaver tissues.

On his doctor's recommendation, Welker waited a month to allow his injury to heal, his swelling to subside, and any excess fluid to reabsorb. In this way, he presented a relatively trauma-free knee for ACL replacement surgery. He opted for a patellar tendon replacement, an option known for maximizing his chances for a complete recovery to top performance.

Welker is a professional athlete - physically and emotionally exceptional. While a motivated person might go to physical therapy twice a week for an hour, and do three sets of ten for each of a dozen or so exercises on the days in between, Welker had the luxury and commitment to work full-time every day with a team of doctors and physical therapists. He went through all the stages of recovery that normal people go through, but more intensely and faster. He was doing cutting drills after four months and was back on the playing field for practice after seven.

Yet despite Welker's early and heroic return to NFL level play, he did not reach peak performance until 18 months after the original injury. The year Welker returned, he had a respectable season with 86 receptions, playing in 15 out of 16 games. The following year, in 2011, Welker had a spectacular year leading the league with 122 catches.

For typical high school or college athletes, the rehab time after an ACL tear is a minimum of nine months, and for many people, a full return to their sport takes a year or more. In the United States, there are more than 150,000 ACL reconstructions every year. That's 150,000 surgeries, and over a million months of physical therapy and rehabilitation. Of course, there are the outlier performances of crazy tough athletes like Los Angeles Chargers' quarterback Philip Rivers who, in 2008, just six days after he tore his ACL, played in the AFC championship game against Tom Brady and the New England Patriots. After losing 21 – 12, Rivers said: "Honestly, it wasn't crazy pain. It kind of buckled a few times in the game, but I really was thankful. Throughout the course of the game, I didn't feel like it hindered me as much as I anticipated." Rivers eventually had surgery and underwent rehab, but he did not miss a game.

It is not uncommon for an athlete to tear his/her ACL and then tear it again. St. Louis Rams star quarterback, hope for the future and Heisman trophy winner, Sam Bradford tore his ACL in 2013, running out of bounds. A star rookie in 2010, Bradford looked like he could lead the Rams to contention, but he was injury prone and suffered the dreaded ACL tear. A year later, looking healthy and performing well after rehab, he reinjured the reconstructed knee when a linebacker rolled onto his locked leg in a low impact collision. Bradford limped off the field. At first nobody thought that he had sustained any serious injury, but later it was confirmed that he had torn his ACL once again. He missed the entire 2014 season but came back strongly in 2015 with the Eagles and in 2016 with the Vikings. In 2017, the wear and tear on his knee after two previous ACL surgeries put him on injured reserve status and he missed the rest of the season. Traded to the Arizona Cardinals in 2018, he was unable to keep a starting quarterback position, and was eventually released, ending his career in the NFL

Professional football has no monopoly on the drama of ACL tears. Just before the all-star break of the 2012-2013 NBA season, the Boston Celtics were struggling at three games under an even record. They had lost six games straight, the last being a double overtime loss to the Atlanta Hawks, a game in which they had been leading by 27 points! The Celtics still had three starting all-star players from their last championship season in 2007-2008 with Kevin Garnett, Paul Pierce, and Rajon Rondo. Their bench was deep, and the Celtics were trying to understand why their chemistry had not yet blended.

Rondo, in particular, was having a career season: he was elected to the NBA all-star team, and led the league with an average of 11 assists per game. In the loss against Atlanta, Rondo scored 16 points, pulled down 10 rebounds, and dished out 11 assists, his fifth *triple-double* of the season. Rondo played 45 minutes in the Atlanta loss, and was slightly injured in the fourth quarter but never left the game. He got bumped badly, stepped awkwardly, but did not fall down, limp, or falter. Indeed, Rondo scored his last basket with 30 seconds left in the game, near the end of the second overtime, nearly 12 minutes after his injury.

The Atlanta loss was Friday night, and the Celtics were due to play the NBA champion Miami Heat on national television at 1:00 PM Sunday afternoon, on January 27, 2013. It was a big game, not only because of the expected national audience, but because Ray Allen was going to play in the Boston Garden for the first time since he left the Celtics a year earlier. Allen, the fourth starter on the Celtics 2008 championship team had chosen to leave the Celtics and sign with Miami for reasons related to his playing time and his contract with the Celtics. When Allen signed with the Heat, there were some hard feelings among the fans and some of the players, including Kevin Garnett (KG). Everyone was speculating how/if KG would interact with Allen, and how the Boston fans would react to Allen's return.

Rondo attended the morning *shootaround* with an ice pack around his hamstring, but the team doctor was suspicious and sent Rondo for an MRI before the game. The focus on Allen, the fans, and Garnett faded quickly when minutes before game time it was announced that Rondo would not play because of a strained knee. How would the struggling Celtics stand up against the champion Heat and their superstar LeBron James, without Rajon Rondo? Rondo was their team leader and the Celtics had no organized offense without him. The Celtics, with Rondo, had lost six games straight against some weak teams, so how could the Celtics compete without Rondo against the world champion Miami Heat?

Nonetheless, the Celtics-Heat game was close and competitive at halftime, with the Celtics playing with renewed spirit. If they could play like this without Rondo, maybe they had a chance for the postseason after all? But at halftime, the announcers dropped a bomb: Rondo did not have a mere sprain. The MRI revealed that he had torn the ACL in his right knee, and would be out for the season. The Celtics problems had just begun.

Meanwhile, the Celtics played the second half of their game against the Heat with even more vigor and heart than the first half, and amazingly, they beat the Heat 100-98 in double overtime. The Celtics went on to win their next six games straight without their start point guard, using a collection of guards to fill in for Rondo, including reserve Leandro Barbosa, known for his speed and quickness.

Interestingly, less than two weeks after Rondo's injury, the Celtics winning streak was broken by the lowly Charlotte Bobcats, perhaps the worst team in the NBA in 2013. In this game, Barbosa suffered a torn ACL after planting his left leg awkwardly on a drive to the basket.

He was carried off the court by his teammates, and like Rondo, was out for the season. Barbosa had surgery and rehabbed the knee, but because of his age (30) and the fear that his speed would not ever be the same, he was unable to get a job with the NBA. He signed with a Brazilian team for a year, and impressed the Golden State Warriors to sign him for a one-year contract in 2014-2105, where he was instrumental in helping them win the NBA championship.

Meanwhile in 2013, the Celtics, plagued by injuries, were unable to maintain their intensity in the playoffs, losing in six games to Carmelo Anthony and the NY Knicks. After the 2013 NBA season, the Celtics championship team disbanded: Coach Doc Rivers left, and Pierce and Garnett were traded. The Celtics were left in rebuilding mode with an injured and rehabbing Rondo, whose future was uncertain.

ACL tears occur primarily in athletic pursuits (or in accidents) where the twisting forces are great enough to cause acute damage. The injury is not restricted just to football or basketball. ACL tears occur in soccer, baseball, skiing, golf, rock climbing, gymnastics, hockey, cheerleading, dance, tennis, and in just about any sport where sharp maneuvers are necessary. Swimming, cycling, and running are the three notable sports that are mostly immune from ACL tears. Nonetheless, if you step awkwardly enough, you can tear your ACL slipping on the ice while picking up the morning paper. A friend of mine, who is not particularly athletic, tore her ACL just this way, proving that casual athletes and even couch potatoes are not immune.

Although a great force is necessary to cause an ACL tear, ACL injuries are not usually the result of contact, as Welker, Revis, Bradford, Rondo, and Barbosa can attest to. Many ACL injuries happen when an athlete plants his foot one way, pivots in another direction, and clumsily loses footing or stumbles while still twisted. Because an ACL tear is not always accompanied by a traumatic collision, some athletes do not immediately realize how badly they are injured; they walk off an ACL injury, mistaking the pain for a bad strain.

Rondo, in particular, had a very casual reaction. He continued playing for 12 minutes after his ACL tear, seemingly unaware of the seriousness of his injury. Over the weekend after his injury, Rondo complained of a sore hamstring, but was otherwise asymptomatic. He never knew that he had torn his ACL in the double overtime loss to Atlanta. When interviewed, Rondo claimed that he never even considered that he might have an ACL tear.

"Could I be walking around like this with a torn ACL? I don't feel that bad," Rondo said. "I don't feel like I have something that serious, but I've never had one [a torn ACL] before. All I know is my leg felt funny." [2] Doc Rivers, the Celtics coach, who had suffered a torn ACL himself years earlier, sympathized with his star point guard:

"I told him I remembered the next day after my [ACL tear] I felt pretty good," Rivers said. "I thought the doctors were wrong." [3]

The ultimate example of a *non-contact* ACL tear is the bizarre, embarrassing, and almost comical case of Detroit Lion's middle linebacker Stephen Tulloch. In 2014, he burst through the Green Bay Packer's defense to sack quarterback Aaron Rodgers, and followed it up with a classic NFL exaggerated and undulating celebration dance. Unfortunately for Tulloch, he tore his ACL as he jerked his knees quickly back and forth. And, if you think that no NFL player would ever make that mistake again, just a few weeks later Lamarr Houston of the Chicago Bears did the exact same thing after sacking New England Patriots' backup quarterback Jimmy Garoppolo, the backup quarterback for Tom Brady in 2014-2016.

---

[2] http://espn.go.com/boston/nba/story/_/id/8888143/rajon-rondo-injury-sends-shockwaves-boston-celtics
[3] ibid

Brady is an example of someone who tore his ACL and came back as strong or better than he had been. Brady tore his ACL in 2008, a year before Welker, in a hard contact injury with Bernard Pollard, the same defensive player that confronted Welker before his non-contact ACL tear. Pollard hit Brady hard in the left knee, and unlike Rondo, Brady knew he was injured for sure; Brady did not get back up. The typical tackles that occur in football or soccer are more than enough force to tear an ACL, especially if the knee is hit while the leg is anchored down and cannot give. Brady missed the rest of the 2008 season but came back in top form in 2009 throwing for 378 yards in his first game back after rehab. Brady played effectively for at least ten more seasons, into his forties. Besides his amazing longevity and toughness, he is arguably the greatest quarterback of all time.

Rajon Rondo is not the only NBA superstar guard whose ACL tear affected his team's chances in the playoffs. The 2012 NBA season was a shortened season of 66 games due to player/management disagreements. Just as it seemed the season would be a complete loss, the two sides came to an understanding, and quickly constructed a "short" season. There was no time for training or pre-season games, and many players were not in top shape due to the time off. For a number of players, the short season resulted in a variety of injuries from back sprains to tendinitis.

Superstar Derrick Rose of the Chicago Bulls was one of those players who had accumulated a number of minor injuries, aches, and pains. Rose, the 2011 MVP (most valuable player) award winner, the Bulls team leader, and its best player, plays hard defense, scores, and runs the Bull's offense. Rose missed 27 games of the shortened 2012 season due to injuries, but the Bulls nonetheless amassed the best record in the NBA with 50 wins and 16 losses, going 18-9 without him. They were an amazing team when Rose was with them, but remained a formidable team even without him. Rose, well rested the week before the playoffs, looked ready to play. The Bulls seemed poised to make a run for the championship as Rose suited up for the first game of the first round of the playoffs against the Philadelphia 76-ers on Saturday, April 28, 2012.

In the NBA, the playoffs are the "second season," where teams pick up the intensity and level of their play. The game is rougher, the defense more tenacious, and the desire to win palpable. The 76-ers were a much weaker team and no match for the Bulls, and as expected, the Bulls were having an easy time of it. Leading 99-87, with 1:25 left in the game, Rose brings up the ball and cuts right, dribbling into the paint, pushing hard off his left leg. He lifts up off both legs, jumping high, pumping, and coming down. Still in rhythm, Rose plants both feet and rises once again, this time looking to shoot. Eight feet from the basket, still in the air, and with the Sixers' defense swarming around him, he dishes the ball off to an open Carlos Boozer. Meanwhile, Rose descends back to earth, and falls to the ground grimacing, grabbing his left knee in pain.

The replay shows that on the second jump there is some "give" in the left knee. It looks as though the force of the jump did not just propel Rose upwards, but also forced his left knee inwards quite a bit. The commentators have seen this before, and they know it may be nothing, or it may be big news. They wonder aloud why Bulls coach Tom Thibadou left Rose in a game that was all but over with less than 90 seconds to play. With a decisive lead late in the game, it is common for coaches to sit their stars, in order to protect them from freak season-ending injuries.

The TNT sportscasters, Kevin Harlan and former NBA 3-point shooting star Reggie Miller, obsess over the replay in slow motion trying to find the exact point where the knee gave way and Rose was injured. They finally identify the second jump and the inward motion of the left knee. Back and forth they analyze the action.

Harlan: "Uh-oh, uh-oh, Rose came down bad on his left foot. See him? Holding on to his knee, holding on to his knee, and down. He was flying and he came down wrong on the left foot. Now whether it was his ankle or his knee, I don't know. You see how he comes down on the *left* leg. Keep an eye on the *left* leg. There. Yep. When he plants it, that's when whatever happened, happened. Let's see here."

Miller: "Yeah. It's before he comes down. It's the plant right there on that left leg."

Harlan: "There was some give. There was some give on that knee and you could see it."

Miller: "Looked like it went in too."

Harlan: "That's what I'm saying."

Rose had torn the ACL in his left knee, his season was over, and the Bulls were moving into four rounds of playoff matches without their leader and star. Fans were heartbroken; pundits second-guessed Coach Thibadou's decision to leave Rose in the game at that point; and experts downgraded the Bulls chances of winning a championship from very high to slim. Indeed, the Bulls did not make it past the first round of the playoffs. They were eliminated by the inferior Philadelphia 76-ers, who were beaten by the Boston Celtics, who were in turn defeated by the Miami Heat, led by LeBron James.

James, perhaps the greatest superstar in the NBA, had yet to prove that he could lead a team to an NBA championship title. Many labeled him a "choker." Indeed, an NBA title was the only accomplishment James was lacking as a basketball player, so he had a lot at stake going into the final championship series in 2012 against Kevin Durant and the Oklahoma Thunder.

Toward the end of the fifth game, with the score very close and the Thunder giving it their last comeback effort, James suddenly fell to the floor and attempted unsuccessfully to hobble to his feet. As he tried once again to stand, he fell a second time and was carried off the

17

court to the bench. Once again, it looked as if LeBron would not be there for his team in the clutch. Not this time. A few minutes later, he came back in and hit a three pointer, putting the game out of reach for good. Then he sat down to watch his team win the game and the 2012 NBA championship.

Fortunately, for the Heat, not every serious looking injury is an ACL tear. LeBron suffered a leg cramp and not the dreaded season-ending ACL injury suffered by Rose and the Bulls. James played a tremendous series, singlehandedly leading his team to victory, and putting a decisive end to his reputation of not being a clutch player. James won the 2012 NBA most valuable player award, while the reigning 2011 MVP award winner, Derrick Rose, was busy in rehab.

After a year of patient and deliberate rehabilitation, Rose returned to the Bulls for the 2013 season but promptly reinjured his knee, and underwent surgery for a torn meniscus, once again missing the rest of the season. The Bulls, led by Joakim Noah, valiantly made it to the 2013 playoffs, but without Rose, they were eliminated in the first round by the Washington Wizards. Rose came back for two more seasons with the Bulls, but repeated meniscus tears necessitated multiple surgeries that bounced him from MVP caliber play to injured reserve status. He continued to play effectively in the NBA as a journeyman role player for the Knicks (2016), Cavaliers (2017), Timberwolves (2018), and Pistons (2019).

More recently Klay Thompson of the Golden State Warriors tore his ACL in the 2019 NBA finals against the Toronto Raptors who won the series in six games, killing the Warriors hopes for a three-peat. Thompson, fouled on a breakaway layup, landed awkwardly on his left foot, fell down and grabbed his left knee in pain. The slow-motion replay showed his left knee buckling inwards with that tell-tale unnatural inward bend, and his leg was unable to bear the weight of his body with his knee not lined up in a straight line. Klay walked off the court to get checked by the doctor, and came back five minutes later making both free-throws, and keeping the right to play the rest of the game in case he was cleared by the doctor. Kevin Durant tore his Achilles tendon earlier in the series, so Thompson's injury left the Warriors critically short of talent. Thompson wasn't cleared to return to the game. Word came back that he was out of the game with an ACL tear and that he will miss the 2020 season. And, KD was picked up the Brooklyn Nets as a free agent. The Warriors dynasty is over.

Major league baseball players are also not immune from the dreaded ACL injury. Mariano Rivera, famed relief pitcher of the New York Yankees, holds the current major league baseball record for career saves with 608, and boasts five World Series rings.

"I always argued he (Rivera) was the best pitcher of all-time, not just the best reliever, but the best pitcher of all-time," said Yankee first baseman Mark Teixeira. Whether or not Teixeira is right, Rivera is certainly one of the most durable pitchers of all-time, pitching effectively into his forties. Nonetheless, an ACL tear can happen to anybody at any time.

Teixeira summed it all up: "Accidents happen. That's all I can say. You can get hurt getting out of bed, literally. You can get hurt doing anything… That's Mo. Part of what makes him great is he's so athletic, and he loves to run around out there and have fun. You can't play this game for 15-plus years without having fun. It was just a tough accident."[4]

Throughout his career prior to each game, the 42 year-old Rivera has shagged fly balls in the outfield for conditioning, fun, and practice. In May 2012, before a game against the Kansas City Royals, Rivera was chasing down a fly ball in Kauffman Stadium. His cleat caught on the grass, his knee buckled, and he fell to the ground grimacing. Manager Joe Girardi said, "My thought was he has a torn ligament, by the way he went down." And, Joe was right. Rivera

---

[4] Dave Skretta article AP

underwent an MRI exam and was diagnosed with a torn ACL and a torn meniscus. The Yankees went on to lose the Royals by a score of 4 to 3. This ended Rivera's season, and at age 42, his major league baseball career might have been over.

Rivera had surgery and underwent a rehabilitation program. He was running again by 2013, eight months after his injury, and he returned to spring training for the MLB 2013 season. Rivera pitched effectively in 2013 and was elected, as usual, to the American League all-star team. When he reached the pitcher's mound for what was to be his last all-star appearance, he received a standing ovation from both dugouts. He won the MVP award in that 2013 MLB all-star game, shutting down the National League batters in the 8th inning on just 16 pitches. Rivera retired at the end the of the 2013 season.

Rehabilitation is the key to a successful return from ACL surgery. Professionals devote themselves fulltime to rehab, and often return close to their pre-injury performance level after months of hard work. There are a number of amazing comebacks from ACL injuries, but perhaps no story exhibits as much heroic perseverance as that of skier Picabo Street. Of all sports, skiing is probably the toughest on an athlete's knees. Street's recovery from knee injury was nothing short of miraculous.

In the years 1995 and 1996, Picabo Street was the most famous skier in the United States, having won two World Cup downhill titles and a gold medal in the World Championship. ESPN considered her the "greatest female speed skier in the world." [5] In December 1996, Street tore the ACL in her left knee during a training run in Vale. Street's ACL was surgically replaced, and she was out for the 1997 season. Her rehab consisted of swimming, volleyball, and more than 10,000 hours on treadmills, Stairmasters, and stationary bikes. Amazingly, she surprised

---

[5] http://www.espn.go.com/classic/biography/s/Street_Picabo.html

everyone by returning to the slopes in 1998 ready to do battle at the Nagano, Japan winter Olympics.

In her last pre-Olympic competition in Are, Sweden, she crashed into a fence at 75 mph and blacked out. She suffered a concussion, but walked away from the accident undaunted and confident. "That crash was a blessing in disguise," she said. "I wondered what would happen when I went down, and I proved to myself I was 100 percent healthy. I took confidence out of that incident. Adversity makes heroes."

Suffering from neck pain and headaches as a result of her crash and concussion, but armed with the knowledge that her ACL replacement was intact and reliable, Street won an Olympic gold medal in the Super G (super giant slalom). After her 1998 Olympic triumph, Street competed at the end of the season in Crans-Montana, Switzerland, where disaster struck. She crashed badly, shattering her left femur in nine places and tearing her other ACL, this time in her *right* knee. This setback resulted in two more years of rehabilitation, but incredibly, at the age of 30, she competed once again in the 2002 Utah Olympics. Unfortunately, she was never able to regain the dominance of her earlier career after this second ACL tear, finishing 16th in the downhill in Salt Lake City, and retiring from professional skiing at age 30.

Street is not the only skier whose career was cut short by an ACL injury. More recently, in February 2013, Lindsay Vonn, the most accomplished female skier is U.S. history, tore her ACL in a crash during the Alpine skiing world championship in Schlamding, Austria.[6] Vonn won the gold medal in the 2010 Olympic woman's downhill, and hoped to repeat that accomplishment in 2014 in Sochi. Unfortunately, after surgery and rehab, she repeatedly reinjured the knee in a number of different accidents, dashing her hopes, and forcing her to pull

---

[6] http://www.today.com/sochi/lindsey-vonn-withdraws-sochi-olympics-my-knee-just-too-unstable-2D11869416

out of the 2014 Sochi games. She is scheduled for further surgery and hopes to be back for the World Championships in Vail in February 2015. The future of Vonn's career is uncertain.

Like Vonn's injury, many ACL tears are memorable events, involving a particular fall, or jump, or hit, along with swelling and pain. However, athletes are used to pain and adversity and sometimes an ACL tear is overlooked as just another minor injury to work through. The next story deals with an ACL tear that was undiagnosed for months.

You may not remember, but the greatest golfer of the last twenty years, Tiger Woods, tore his ACL. The reason you might not remember is because he himself was unaware of the tear. In April 2008, in a hard-fought battle, Woods, a previous four-time winner of the Masters tournament, had come in second place, three strokes behind Trevor Immelman of South Africa, who won with a score of eight under par. When Woods was at the top of his game, it was news when he did *not* win a closely fought tournament. Against Immelman, something seemed to bother him, and it turned out to be a torn meniscus and a previously undiagnosed ACL tear. The official story is that Tiger Woods tore his ACL jogging in 2007. No other details are known, and neither Woods, nor anyone else, seems to have been aware of the torn ligament until after the 2008 Masters, when he underwent arthroscopic surgery to repair the torn meniscus.

After learning of the ACL tear, Woods decided to delay any treatment until after the US Open. He went on to win the 2008 US Open on a 19th hole playoff, limping through much of the round, sometimes using his club as a cane. After his victory, Woods took off the rest of the season and scheduled surgery.

Joseph Bosco, M.D., an orthopedic surgeon at New York University and spokesman for the American Academy of Orthopaedic Surgeons, said "The natural history of anterior cruciate ligaments treated non-operatively is that patients go on to develop cartilage damage," implying

22

that Woods almost surely damaged his meniscus and other cartilage in his knee by playing actively for over a year on the torn ACL. Dr. Bosco added that although nobody who has ACL reconstruction ever again has a "normal knee," 90% of professionals resume their careers after surgical replacement and 6-12 months of rehab. Further, he expects Woods not merely to return to golf, but to dominate the sport like he did before his ACL tear.[7]

In November 2009, less than a year after Tiger's return from physical rehab to the tour, and before anyone expected that he would regain his previous dominance, Woods suddenly found himself saddled with far more difficult problems. A suspicious car accident, revelation of infidelities, and the subsequent break-up of his marriage required an emotional rehabilitation that proved even more difficult than the physical rehab.

Woods had moments of brilliance since his ACL tear, including the US Open win before his surgery, but since his replacement surgery, it looked like he might never return to his previous level of play and dominance of the sport. Then in 2019, he won the Masters – an amazing comeback from one of the greatest golfers of all time.

Although some athletes make heroically fast returns from rehab after an ACL tear, even the dedication and athleticism of the best athletes cannot bring a player back sooner than six months. At the start of the 1997 NFL season, Jerry Rice, the hall-of-fame wide receiver, had played 189 consecutive games - the iron man of football. Rice is known for his work ethic and dedication to the game. He holds records for most career receptions, receiving yards, and touchdowns. He has scored a touchdown in four different super bowls, and is considered the greatest route runner in NFL history. He is fast, strong, and agile; if anyone could come back from ACL surgery early, it would be him.

---

[7] http://www.medpagetoday.com/Surgery/Orthopedics/9870

While running a reverse against Tampa Bay in the opening game of the season, Rice was pulled down by his facemask, resulting in a penalty against the opposing team and a torn ACL for Rice. Only 14 weeks later that same season, he returned to the playing field against the orders of his doctors, insisting on full contact scrimmage practice only three months after ACL replacement surgery. Although his rehab had gone perfectly and Rice seemed to be in great shape, things did not go so well for him on the field.

Rice quickly caught a pass for a touchdown, landed on the ground, and cracked the patella where the graft for his ACL replacement had been harvested. Even Jerry Rice cannot fool with Mother Nature; he played only two games in the 1997 season. Amazingly, Rice subsequently made a full recovery and was back in 1998 with a stellar season.

Unfortunately, some athletes never return to their former sports after ACL recovery, especially if their injury was pre-1980, when surgical techniques were not yet as effective as they are today. As athletes continue to push themselves harder and compete more intensely, ACL injuries occur more often. Surgeons are always looking for more effective ways to allow athletes to return to their sports more quickly, perform at a level at least as good as pre-injury, and avoid premature retirement.

One of the quickest and successful ACL recoveries in recent years is that of Adrian Peterson, a running back for the Minnesota Vikings, and probably the best running back in the NFL. Peterson tore his ACL at the end of the 2011 season on Christmas Eve, after planting his leg and being tackled hard. He underwent surgery immediately, committed to rehab fervently, and was back for the 2012 season, just nine months after his injury.

Amazingly, he had a career season. He rushed for over 2000 yards, just short of the NFL single season record held by Eric Dickerson, and won the NFL 2012 MVP award. Peterson is the poster child for ACL surgery recovery, and serves as a motivating influence for other athletes. He attributes his amazing recovery to hard work and commitment.

"It's really all about how you approach the recovery... There are a lot of guys that really talk about coming back and recovering from a serious injury but don't really put the work in to do it. Mentally, just believing that you're going to come back and you're going to be better, that's a huge part of it. That sounds cliché. That sounds simple, but you have to believe it in order to accomplish it. You've really got to put the work in behind it as well."[8]

In retrospect, it is astounding that Rice tried to return to NFL competition a mere three months after surgery, when Peterson, the king of ACL recovery, took nine. To have expected to duplicate Peterson's accomplishment in a third the time was impossible even for Jerry Rice, who was every bit as committed as Adrian Peterson.

Interviewed recently about NFL star Adrian Peterson's ACL rehabilitation schedule, Rice recommended patience. "I thought I was invincible. I felt I did all the work and it was time for me to get back on that football field. But if I had to do it all over again, I would take more time to heal up, then come back."

An even more amazing recovery than Peterson is that of Canadian freestyle skier Kaya Turski. In August 2013, Kaya was perfecting a difficult 720-degree rotation trick, and blew out her ACL when she hit the snow a half-rotation early. "I was so lost in the air... When I hit the ground still rotating, I felt my ACL go. I knew I blew it. I know what it feels like." [9] Indeed, Turski had previously torn both ACLs and repaired each with her own hamstring grafts. With

[8] http://www.washingtontimes.com/blog/redskins-watch/2013/feb/5/adrian-petersons-advice-rg3-recovering-acl-surgery/#ixzz2K8D7KLGx
[9] http://xgames.espn.go.com/skiing/article/10195857/kaya-turski-bouncing-back-revolutionary-knee-surgery

less than six months left until the Sochi Olympics, she did not have nine months available for the standard ACL replacement rehabilitation. The third time was not a charm for Turski.

There is usually no shortcut to the yearlong rehab necessary after ACL-replacement surgery; however, Turski was determined not to give up hope. She learned that an artificial ACL replacement would speed up recovery time greatly. Indeed, a synthetic replacement requires no time to grow to full strength and leaves no secondary weaknesses from the harvest site. Unfortunately, over the long term, these synthetic polyester replacements, known as LARS ligaments, are well known to fray and fail under stress. That is, with a LARS replacement, Kaya might be able to compete in Sochi, but her knee might soon afterwards be unstable again. Furthermore, because of her previous ACL replacements, the tunnels in the bones where the synthetic replacement ACL would be affixed were too big for a LARS ligament.

The Canadian Alpine ski team orthopedic surgeon, Brian Litchfield, suggested an interesting compromise: wrapping a LARS ligament inside an allograft (human cadaver tissue). This combination had the advantage of fast rehabilitation without the long-term risks of graft failure. The allograft would grow stronger with time and handle any stress that the LARS ligament might not. And, the allograft/synthetic combo would fill her predrilled tunnels more effectively.

Turski underwent the experimental surgery, and had one of the most amazing ACL recoveries in history. She was back on skis three months later in November 2013, and won a gold medal in the women's Ski Slopestyle at the Aspen X-games in January 2014. A month after the X-games, and only six months after surgery, she was ready to compete at the Sochi Olympics. Unfortunately, she contracted a nasty virus and tumbled in her preliminary runs dislocating her shoulder. Popping her shoulder back into place, she continued to compete but did not make the finals, coming in 19th out of 22 competitors.

In extremely rare cases following an ACL tear, an athlete successfully returns to his/her sport without surgery. DeJuan Blair plays power forward in the NBA. He played four seasons for the San Antonio Spurs averaging about 8 points and 5 rebounds per game, and in 2013, he signed with the Dallas Mavericks. Blair is an anomaly. He tore both ACLs in high school, but never had them surgically replaced. Instead, the torn ligaments slowly deteriorated and disappeared. Normally, without an ACL, the knee is unstable, and can separate under the stress of strong twists and turns. Instability makes an athlete lose confidence, develop compensating poor form, and can result in further injuries to cartilage. Somehow, Blair's quadriceps, hamstrings, and other ligaments and tendons effectively do the job of his missing ACLs. Blair seems to have slowly adapted his form and strengthened the necessary muscles while his ACLs gradually atrophied. Without ACLs, it is usually impossible for an athlete to play a sport that requires cuts and twists… but Blair seems to be an exception.

For almost all athletes, returning to their sports means surgery. Unfortunately, surgery takes its toll on the body. The only way to recover successfully from ACL replacement surgery is to patiently work very hard over a long period of time. The physical challenge, however, is not necessarily as hard as the emotional challenge. Athletes tend to be a motivated and hard-working bunch, but they are not used to being handicapped; and they are not accustomed to progressing slowly. Their broken bodies can shake their usual confidence, competence, and success.

The beautiful and athletic Malaysian actress and dancer Michelle Yeoh, who played Wai Lin in the 1997 James Bond film *Tomorrow Never Dies*, insists on doing her own stunts and

27

fight scenes. In 2000, she starred in the award-winning *Crouching Tiger, Hidden Dragon*, where she tore her ACL during the filming. She describes the injury:

"The first action sequence was very intensive. I was doing a forward jump quick that I've done thousands of times, but I had a mishap landing... I thought 'I'm fine,' ... but I knew it was bad when I turned left, and my leg kept swinging right."

After surgery, physical therapy, and rehab, Yeoh is back to her craft, but admits "You never get all the way back to what it was."

Every athlete reacts differently to the challenges posed by recovery from ACL replacement. The professional athletes discussed here constitute a spectrum, but there are dozens of other professional athletes who have torn their ACLs. Here is a list, not meant to be complete, that might contain some of your favorites:[10]

Basketball: Lou Williams, Jason Smith, Al Harrington, Ricky Rubio, David West, Jamal Crawford, Kendrick Perkins, Bernard King, Rajon Rondo, Derek Rose, DeJuan Blair, Danilo Gallinari, Dante Exum, Klay Thompson, DeMarcus Cousins.

Football: Greg Camarillo, Tyler Roehl, Deion Branch, Terrell Owens, Kris Jenkins, Adrian Peterson, Tom Brady, Wes Welker, Jerry Rice, Bryan Bulaga, Darrelle Revis, Sam Bradford, Rob Gronkowski, Jeremy Maclin, Dan Koppen, Jason Phillips, Stephen Tulloch, Stevan Ridley, Lamarr Houston, Carlson Palmer, Dion Lewis, Justin Houston, Julian Edelman.

Soccer: Frankie Hejuk, Michael Owen, Megan Rapinoe, Mikel Arteta, Robert Pires, Roberto Baggio, Alessandro Del Piero, Ruud van Nistelrooy, Alan Shearer

Hockey: Andrew Brunette, Alex Galchenyuk, Pavel Bure, Marek Svatos, Robby Fabbri

---

[1010] http://yeskneecan.com/2009/06/16/recent-famous-athletes-w-torn-acls/ (kneegeeks)

Baseball:	Chipper Jones, Victor Martinez, Lance Berkman, Yovani Gallardo, Mariano Rivera, Kyle Schwarber
Gymnastics:	Shawn Johnson, Aliya Mustafina
Skiing:	Picabo Street, Lindsay Vonn, Kaya Turski, Andrea Limbacher
Golf:	Tiger Woods
Tennis:	Mary Pierce
Dance:	Michelle Yeo, Pamela Swaney

American Ninja Warrior: Angela Gargano, Drew Drechsel, Erica Cook

And, the list grows all the time. Listen to the sports news regularly and you are sure to hear of the next unfortunate celebrity athlete.

So if you've torn your ACL, you are in good company. Now start reading and learn how to best prepare for the decisions you will need to make on the long road to recovery.

Chapter 2 – Basic Anatomy of the Knee

"The knee bone connected to the thigh bone"

Dem Dry Bones – a spiritual song

The knee is the largest joint in the human body consisting of a complex combination of bones, cartilage (menisci), ligaments, muscles, and tendons. Together these parts allow smooth movement, shock absorption, quick acceleration, and sharp but stable changes in direction.

Bones:

Bones are hard strong and light structures that give our body its rigidity. They have good blood flow and heal well. The knee is the juncture of your thighbone, called the femur, and the two lower bones of the leg, the tibia and the fibula. The *femur* is an impressive bone – the largest in your body. It runs from your hip to the knee. At the knee it bulges into two bumps with a cleavage shaped indentation in between.

From the lower end of your leg, two bones come up from your ankle to meet the femur at the knee, one on the outside and one on the inside. The terms inside and outside are intuitive. To be clear, when facing forward, the outside of your knee refers to the right side of the right knee and the left side of the left knee, while the inside of your knee refers to the left side of the right knee and the right side of the left knee.

Of the two bones in the lower leg that meet the femur, the *fibula*, thinner and smaller, is on the outside; the *tibia*, thicker and larger, is on the inside. The femur sits directly on top of the tibia. The fibula is situated toward the outside corner of the femur, see figure below. The *patella,* your kneecap, covers the cleavage of your femur and its junction with the tibia and fibula. The patella protects the joint from impact from the front.

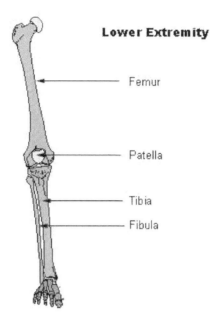

Lower Extremity

— Femur

— Patella

— Tibia

— Fibula

The Bones of your Leg: the Femur, Tibia, Fibula, and Patella.

Ligaments:

A ligament is a fibrous, strong, and slightly stretchy white/gray colored tissue that connects bone to bone. Unlike bones, ligaments do not have good blood supply and are slow to heal when torn or injured. A partially torn ligament can take months or years to heal completely, and a completely torn ligament sometimes never heals.

Four ligaments hold the three bones at the knee joint together and allow for stable movement: MCL, LCL, PCL, and ACL. Two of the ligaments, the MCL and LCL, are at the sides of the knee and prevent the knee from moving too much laterally. The two other ligaments, the PCL and ACL, are in the center (or middle) of the knee, and cross each other like an X.

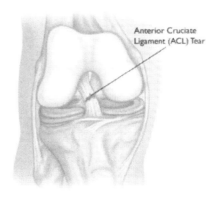

The right knee from the front – showing the four ligaments in pink.[11]

MCL: The *medial collateral ligament* is on the inside of the knee, connecting the femur to the tibia. The MCL prevents the knee from bowing inward too much.

LCL: The *lateral collateral ligament* is on the outside, connecting the femur to the fibula. The LCL prevents the knee from bowing outward too much.

PCL: The *posterior cruciate ligament* runs at an angle from the back inside half of the femur to the back outside half of the tibia. The PCL is about the thickness of a pinky and stops the tibia from moving backwards with respect to the femur. The PCL is not injured as commonly as the ACL in part because it is stronger.

ACL: The *anterior cruciate ligament* runs at an angle from the front outside half of the femur to the front inside half of the tibia, crossing in front of the PCL. The ACL is thinner and less strong than the PCL. The ACL prevents the tibia from moving too far forward with respect to the femur.

The need to keep the tibia from moving too far forward or backward with respect to the femur is mainly due to side-to-side cutting and pivoting motions. When a person

---

[11] http://orthoinfo.aaos.org/topic.cfm?topic=A00297

anchors their foot and swivels his/her hip violently, turning the knee sharply in a different direction from the direction of the pointed foot, the torque from the upper body pulls the femur away from the tibia. The cruciate ligaments (PCL and ACL) keep these bones together through the common but violent rotations of many sports. If all we did was run in a straight line, cycle, or swim, we might very well do fine without our cruciate ligaments. It is primarily twisting motions that generate the forces that stress the cruciate ligaments.

Knee Joint Capsule: The joint capsule is a thick ligament-like structure that surrounds the entire knee. Inside this capsule is a membrane known as the synovial membrane, which provides nourishment to all the surrounding tissue and structures. The capsule is surrounded and strengthened by the MCL and LCL.

ALL: Surprisingly, even today new anatomical structures in the knee are identified and discovered. In 2013, Dr. Claes and other knee surgeons from the University Hospital Leuven in Belgium[12] published a paper in the Journal of Anatomy describing a new ligament called the anterolateral ligament (ALL). Motivated by a number of cases where ACL replacement surgery left patients with unstable knees, Dr. Claes and his colleagues wondered if there might not be another structure that could sustain a destabilizing injury. Indeed, in 1879, a French surgeon named Paul Segond suggested that there might be an additional ligament besides the four major knee ligaments (LCL, MCL, PCL, and ACL). He noticed a fibrous band of tissue on the outside of the knee connecting the femur to the tibia, which seemed to help to stabilize the knee and keep it from collapsing inward. Dr. Segond did not name this structure, nor

---

[12] http://well.blogs.nytimes.com/2013/11/13/a-surprising-discovery-a-new-knee-ligament/

did his paper receive much attention, perhaps because it seems like part of a large fascia called the iliotibial band, (see Fasciae, below). Yet, more than 130 years later, after dissecting dozens of cadaver knees, Dr. Claes discovered a ligament, clearly distinct from the iliotibial band, in a location very much like the one described by Dr. Segond. The ligament was in a position that made it vulnerable to damage whenever the ACL might be damaged. Dr. Claes hypothesizes that patients who experience unstable knees after ACL replacement surgery may have damaged ALLs. Whether a damaged ALL heals on its own, or what kinds of ALL repair might be possible are areas of future research.

Muscles:

Muscles are red tissues that contract and allow movement. The strength of muscles varies depending on their purpose from small muscles in your eye that allow a flirty wink, to the massive muscles in your thigh that let you run and jump. Muscles have excellent blood supply, and heal extremely well and relatively quickly. Small micro-tears in muscles occur normally after hard exercise. You know you have these when you feel sore after a good workout, or perhaps when you overdid it a little. These kinds of tears heal in a matter of 2-3 days and the healing makes the muscle larger and stronger. More serious ruptures, tears, or "pulls," can take weeks to months to heal depending on the degree or severity of the tear. However, regardless of healing time, muscles heal well.

The major muscles related to the knee are the quadriceps and the hamstrings. They are crucial for running, jumping, squatting, and extending the knee. The quadriceps muscle (quads), located at the front of your leg, is really a collection of four muscles. The hamstrings, consisting of a group of three muscles are the opposing muscles at the back of your leg.

When you contract your quads to extend your knee, your hamstrings act in opposition to provide stability. If your quads are much stronger than your hamstrings, the forceful contraction of your quads may be too strong for your hamstrings to control, causing damage to your joints, muscles, or ligaments. Weak hamstrings also fatigue more quickly causing a greater strength imbalance and possibly worse injuries. It is important to maintain balance in the strength of your hamstrings and quads.

Normally the quads are stronger than the hamstrings, but the difference in their strengths can vary a great deal. The ratio of quad strength to hamstring strength ranges from as low as 5:4 to as great as 2:1. You don't want a big imbalance. To avoid knee injury many therapists and trainers recommend keeping the quad to hamstring ratio no greater than 4:3.

Women generally have less strength than men in their quads and hamstrings. Older people also tend to have less strength in both muscle groups. However, besides lower strength, women tend also to have a greater imbalance of strength, while older men maintain similar strength ratios throughout their lives. Some think that this imbalance is one of the reasons women are more prone to ACL injuries.[13]

Tendons:

Tendons are like ligaments except that they connect muscle to bone, rather than bone to bone. Tendons are redder the closer they are to muscle and more gray/white as they approach bone. The closer to the bone, the less blood supply and the weaker the tendon's ability to heal. Severe tears in a tendon may require surgery, but small tears often heal on their own given enough time. The important thing with tendons is not to

---

[13] http://www.livestrong.com/article/442551-hamstrings-vs-quads/#ixzz20LWAA5eT

reinjure them while they are healing, because this can result in chronically swollen tendons and painful tendinitis.

At the bottom of the quadriceps muscle there is the *quadriceps tendon*, which attaches the massive quadriceps muscle to the top of the patella. The bottom of the patella is connected to the tibia by the *patellar tendon*. Technically, the patellar tendon is a ligament because it connects bone to bone, but functionally it is the continuation of the quadriceps tendon, so it usually called the patellar tendon rather than the patellar ligament.

The patellar tendon is the final anchor of the quadriceps muscle to the tibia, which allows the quadriceps to extend and straighten the knee for running, jumping, and kicking. The patellar tendon is about an inch wide and three inches long. Harvesting the middle third is one of the main options for replacing a torn ACL. This piece of tissue, approximately 1 cm by 3.5 cm, without the bones on each end, mirrors the shape and size of the original ACL very closely. Other choices for *autografts* (where the replacement tissue comes from the patient) include tendons in the hamstring.

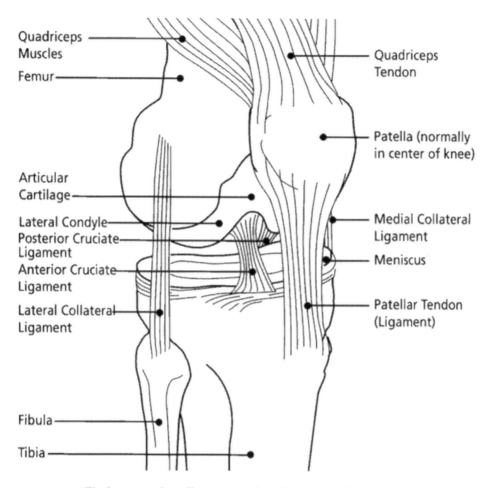

Quadriceps Muscles

Femur

Articular Cartilage

Lateral Condyle

Posterior Cruciate Ligament

Anterior Cruciate Ligament

Lateral Collateral Ligament

Fibula

Tibia

Quadriceps Tendon

Patella (normally in center of knee)

Medial Collateral Ligament

Meniscus

Patellar Tendon (Ligament)

The bones, tendons, ligaments, and cartilage in your knee

Bursae:

These are a dozen or so thin-walled synovial fluid filled sacs that interact with the knee to minimize friction as the various bones, cartilage, and ligaments rub over one another. After an injury, one or more of these may burst causing swelling and pain. After rest, the fluid is reabsorbed and the bursa can grow back effectively. Bursae are rarely the objects of surgery.

Fasciae:

Fasciae are connective tissue much like tendons or ligaments, but whereas tendons connect bone to muscle, and ligaments connect bone to bone, fasciae surround muscles or other structures. Fasciae are the webs of the body; they keep everything in the right place and allow muscles to operate efficiently and smoothly. Injuries to fasciae can cause a significant loss of performance in recreational athletes, and can contribute to secondary disorders, like lower back or hip pain.

A major fascia that helps stabilize the knee during running is called the iliotibial band. This long fibrous fascia runs along the outer thigh from the pelvis to just below the outer side of the knee. This fascia is rarely injured in an ACL tear.

Cartilage and Menisci:

The remaining pieces of the knee called menisci are made of cartilage, a substance with a texture like your ears and nose. The menisci act like shock absorbers every time the femur slams into the tibia. Two menisci sit on top of the tibia covering it with a cartilage cushion. The medial meniscus covers the inside half of the tibia while the lateral meniscus covers the outer half. The medial meniscus is connected to the MCL while the lateral meniscus floats freely from the LCL. This difference increases the chances of medial meniscal tears.

There is also cartilage on the bottom of the femur. A common knee injury is a tear in one or both of the tibial menisci. This often accompanies a torn ACL as the unstable knee moves violently around and through the shock-absorbing menisci.

When I began my rehab and physical therapy I met a guy a little younger than me who was very athletic and had played catcher in college level baseball. He had worn out the articular cartilage at the bottom of his femur by repeated kneeling and squatting. Cartilage does not grow back, and artificial cartilage is not usually effective, so amazingly the doctors were trying to re-grow his cartilage. Using small pieces of his own tissue-harvested months earlier and then grown and nourished in the lab, they implanted the new growth onto the bottom of his femur. He had a long road of rehab ahead (18 months) until full recovery, but he looked forward to normal activity including skiing among other knee-intensive sports. I did not follow up to see how he was doing 18 months later, but these techniques are in their infancy, and we have years of experimenting and improvement to come.

ACL surgery today is more advanced and less experimental than cartilage replacement surgery, but this was not the case twenty-five years ago. Surgery for ACL replacement 25 years ago was "open" rather than arthroscopic. Open knee surgery is like the way you dissected a frog in high school biology. The knee is sliced completely open to see what you are doing – two horizontal incisions at the top and bottom, and one vertical incision connecting the midpoints of the horizontal incisions. The two resulting flaps are opened up revealing the knee underneath. This kind of surgery is more traumatic and causes more pain and damage. Nowadays, *arthroscopic* surgery is much less invasive with procedures being done through small holes using scopes to see what is going on.

The catcher told me that 25 years earlier he completely tore his ACL playing baseball. At the time, surgical techniques were not as advanced and outcomes not as good, so instead of undergoing the risks of surgery, he used a brace and played the rest of the season. In the end, he never underwent surgery for his torn ACL. Ten years later he had an MRI for an unrelated injury and the films revealed that his stub of an ACL had reattached itself. This was confirmed diagnostically with the Lachman test, a manipulation of the leg used to measure the knee's stability.

Generally, complete tears of the ACL do not spontaneously heal themselves. Although some people seem to be able to function normally without an ACL, it is extremely rare for a torn ACL to grow back together. Whether this man's ACL had been completely torn is impossible to say. Mild and partial ACL tears can heal themselves, so perhaps that explains his story.

Chapter 3 – One Athlete's Tale

"A sailing trip to Great Misery Island? Sure, sounds like fun."

Shai Simonson

This is my story: from the accident through the surgery. Infused into this tale is everything he learned about ACL tears as he went through the process of discovering the injury, deciding whether or not to have surgery, and finally undergoing the ACL replacement procedure. The post-surgery rehab piece is the focus of Chapter 5.

Reading my story will teach you a lot about ACL tears, the details of the surgery, and the issues important in making an informed decision about how to treat your injury. There are many ways to tear one's ACL, and my tale is just one but it is typical. Chapter 6 contains a large variety of other athlete's stories, and you might find someone there who had an experience more directly similar to your own.

A Sailing Trip

I am a very typical middle-age guy who likes to stay fit. I commute to work by bike; I like to hike, and I play ultimate Frisbee and disc golf. Sometimes I swim, run, or play basketball. I do enough to stay in shape; I am active but I am not particularly athletic. I could never run a sub seven-minute mile, never ran more than 9 miles at a time, my swimming form is horrendous - more than a half a mile puts me in danger of drowning, and I spent most of high school on the bench of my synagogue's basketball team. Rather than swimming, cycling, and running, my kind of triathlon is watching TV, snacking, and napping. Nonetheless, you don't need to be a world-class athlete to tear your ACL. Tearing your ACL can happen to anyone, anytime, and it is always an unwelcome surprise. I hope that my experience will help you learn about this devastating injury through an average patient's perspective. Here is my story.

In June of 2011, I was out sailing with friends off the shore of Salem, MA. Before heading out to open ocean, we planned to visit Great Misery Island, a mixed habitat of forest, small meadows, and rocky shores. It is one of many reservations in Massachusetts administered by The Trustees of Reservations. The description in their brochure reads:

> *The ruins of an early-20th-century resort reveal that this offshore retreat was a haven for leisure and recreation a century ago. And the diversity of habitats – groves of aspen, open meadows, rugged and rocky shorelines – adds to the wild beauty of the islands. More than two miles of trails at Great Misery Island lead you to spectacular overlooks, stony beaches, and grassy fields.*

Four of us set sail: two middle-aged friends, myself, and my oldest son who was 19. We anchored the sailboat and took the dinghy, two at a time, to a natural landing spot on the beach. The island is indeed a charming place with beaches, small ponds and forests, nature and hiking trails, and old ruins. We scouted about, picked up seashells, climbed trees, and took pictures. It was a breezy beautiful summer afternoon and we started down one of the hiking trails.

The trail winds in and out of the woods, at times following the shore, and it eventually climbs back for good toward the center of the island. Choosing not to follow the trail back to the center of the island, I continued walking along the rocky shore. My two friends were not as interested as I was in picking a path through and around the riprap and jumble of boulders that formed this part of the island's shore, so they followed the trail back to our beach landing spot. My son followed me, a few hundred feet behind, picking his own path through the rocks.

42

Our family hikes a lot, and we like scrambling. The White Mountains in New Hampshire has been an annual trip of ours for 15 years, and we have hiked dozens of different trails in the Presidential Range, Franconia Notch, Crawford Notch, and the Pemigewasset Wilderness. The highest peak in the Whites, and in the northeast United States, is Mount Washington, at 6288 feet. I've been up and down Mount Washington more than a dozen times, my favorite way up being the steep scramble through Huntington Ravine. We've hiked in the Rockies, the Sierra Nevada, the Cascades, and around Mont Blanc in the Alps. We've done Zion, Bryce, Yosemite, Kings Canyon, Mount Rainier, Mount St. Helens, Rocky Mountain National Park, the Grand Canyon, and many other lesser known, but equally stunning places, all over the country and the world.

When I was in college I used to run and I liked to climb. There was a building under construction near the school that rose up from the cliffs of Morningside Heights overlooking the northwest corner of Central Park in Manhattan. After a 4-mile run through the Upper West Side, my friend Michael and I ran back to my dorm, grabbed his SLR camera, snuck into the construction site, and climbed through the girders and half-completed staircases until we got to the roof of the building. There was a ten-foot high air conditioning housing atop the roof and we scampered up. The view was spectacular, and he snapped this photograph. My knees were young and strong, and I am fortunate that they remained that way as I age. I rarely need to pop Ibuprofens before or after long hikes.

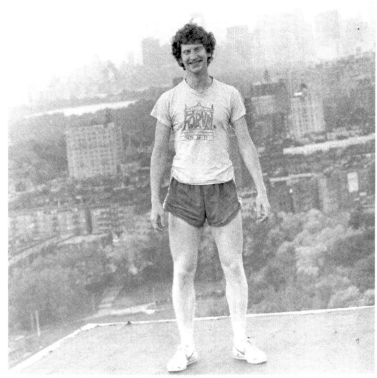

New York – Columbia University – 1979 – overlooking Central Park

As I moved into my late middle years, I recruited different hiking buddies to join me as we checked off our bucket list of day hikes one by one, including a spectacular and famous hike up Half Dome in Yosemite, which finishes with a 400-foot climb over the back of the dome using cables to avoid a fatal fall. My friend Dean and I climbed Half Dome and posed for a scary looking picture on the famous "visor," a rock jutting out off the side of the cliff over a 2000-foot drop. The picture is scarier than it looks – I don't take real risks. The rock we were standing on was quite large and flat, and the edge of the cliff was not too close.

Hiking is a passion and a joy for me. I am sure-footed, experienced, and in reasonable shape. I have never had a serious hiking accident, and I never expected to injure my knee while hiking.

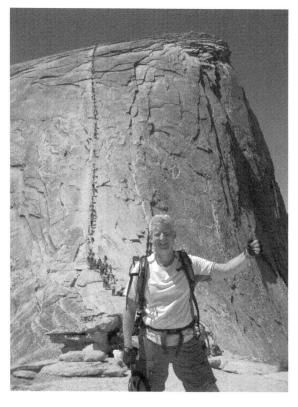

The last 400 feet of the famous Half Dome hike in Yosemite National Park, Summer 2010.

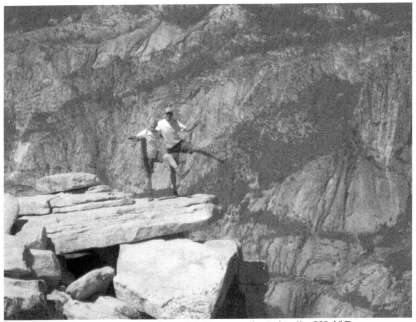
Yosemite 2010 - Balancing with Dean on the "visor" of Half Dome

Meanwhile, back at Great Misery Island, I hurried around the island's rocky shore to join up with my friends, who were probably waiting for me back at the beach. At one point, it was not obvious how to keep bounding from one rock to the next. I got stuck but had no intention of retracing my steps all the way back having come this far. After looking around, it seemed that a scramble down to a short ledge, a little jump from the ledge to the water, followed by a climb back up to another boulder, would send me hopping along. My son was still too far back for me to ask his opinion, but instead of waiting or thinking any further, I pushed ahead with my plan. It wasn't really a bad plan. If I had been just a little more careful, it might have even been a good one.

I stepped down from the boulder with my right foot to a small foothold that I estimated was two or three feet below me. I did not watch where my foot was going because I assumed, incorrectly, that the area around the foothold was flat, and even if the step were a longer reach than I had estimated, the worst-case scenario would be a need for a little stretch. I had done things like this a thousand times, and I was not all that concerned. I expected my toe to be pointed parallel to the slope of the rocks with the outside of my foot facing downward toward the ocean.

My foot went down but did not land when I expected it to, so I stretched the leg out completely and let my weight go. If I did not feel the rock, I expected to jump down another foot or so if necessary, but there was no need to jump. With all my weight now coming down on my right leg, my foot landed on the ledge. Unfortunately, I had been wrong about the ledge – rather than flat, the ledge bent downwards at a 50-degree angle. To avoid tumbling off the ledge and banging my head, I pressed hard and down with my right foot to try and stick the landing.

My weight pushed my knee outward as though I were doing the Charleston on one leg. Ouch! Then as my body followed and my weight came off the other leg, my landing leg straightened out and the knee snapped back the other way, bowing sharply inward. Snap, crackle, pop! Ouch again. Then my right hip landed hard on the rock and broke my fall. My head was intact and I could still think. I just wasn't sure if I could still walk.

My first thought was what an idiot I am, and how I ruined the rest of my summer with one careless step. I switched quickly to a more productive line of thinking and to some practical questions. How was I going to get back to the beach and my buddies if I had trashed my leg? Would my son find me or walk right by me? Meanwhile, hyperventilating in mild panic and desperately trying to catch my breath, I attempted to evaluate my condition and figure out how to deal with this situation.

I tried to be calm and sat back on the rock. I waved nonchalantly in the distance at a recreational sailboat, acting as though I was enjoying the view, rather than stuck in a normally inaccessible part of the shoreline. When I got my wind back, I noted a huge painful bruise on my right hip and upper thigh, and stood up. It hurt to stand but not too badly. It looked like I would be okay. As a young man in my twenties, I had broken a leg playing softball, so I knew what a broken bone felt like, and this was not that. There was a little pain and swelling now, but I could definitely walk it off. For sure I would be okay.

Just around this time, my son came along behind me, asked if I was all right and why I did not wait for him. He has a knack for asking the right questions. Why indeed? We scrambled back together, and when we met up with my buddies at the beach, I quickly walked into the cold ocean to "ice" the leg. That felt good, and although I had some pain, a bad thigh bruise, and a little limp, my summer was not going to be wrecked by my carelessness. Back in the boat, I napped with my leg raised while everybody else sailed and sunned.

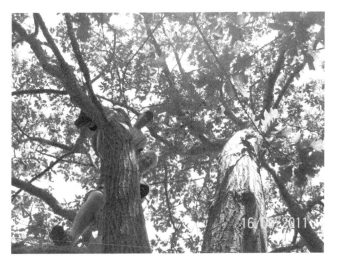

Climbing a tree on Great Misery Island minutes before my accident

I did not sleep so well that night, but two days later I was cycling, in four days I was dancing at a wedding, and after a week, the rainbow colors of my bruise had disappeared. I was pretty sure I was fine, but to be safe, I contacted my doctor who ordered an X-ray. Turns out I hadn't broken anything – no surprise there. The X-ray did indicate some "water on the knee," i.e., excess fluid, but that was normal after an injury; fluid is often caused by small tears of blood vessels.

My discomfort was mostly in the thigh bruise with some minor pain on both sides of the knee, where the MCL (medial collateral ligament) and LCL (lateral collateral ligament) are located. If anything had happened on the island, it seemed like the worst might be some sprained ligaments. After some *googling* around, I learned that minor sprains of the MCL and LCL heal on their own, so I went about my usual business and promised my doctor to keep him informed in case things did not improve.

I spent the next two months doing a lot of summer cycling. I rode two to three hours a day (between 30 and 50 miles) and by the end of the summer my knee felt 100%. My pain was all gone, I had dropped ten pounds, and I had forgotten completely about Great Misery Island.

There was one strange thing that happened to me after the fall on Great Misery Island that I dismissed at the time as unimportant; I only realized its significance months later. I went disc golfing a few days after the injury. Disc golfing is a sport where you throw Frisbees at targets and count the throws. It is a great sport requiring technique, planning, strength, and flexibility. A good throw requires an accelerating rotation of the hips followed by the shoulders and then the arm and wrist. The disc snaps out of the fingers and the thrower's body looks a little like a whip cracking. An athletic beginner can throw the disc about two hundred feet, while a top professional player (yes there are professional disc golf players, see http://pdga.com) routinely throws 400 to 500 feet. I can throw 300 feet and I spend a lot of time trying to improve my strength, flexibility, and technique.

Two days after my fall on Great Misery Island, I was in the field at Borderland State Park practicing my drives, and I took a long pull on the disc, rotating hard through the pull. Strangely, I fell down in the middle of the throw feeling as though my leg just gave out from under me. This had never happened to me before. I continued practicing with a little less enthusiasm (translation: less rotation speed) and everything seemed fine. I chalked up the fall to my poor form and stumbling clumsy approach. Once again I was wrong - not about the poor form and clumsy approach, but about why I fell down. Although I did not know it at the time, the giving out of my knee was very significant. Indeed, this knee instability would reappear three months later at the end of the summer.

Lean, strong, and pain-free by summer's end, I was cycling daily and playing disc golf almost as often without any concerns or difficulties. It was three months after my injury, and I met some friends for a round of disc golf at the Borderland Disc Golf Course in Easton, MA. As I stepped up to drive the 6th hole, one of the longer open holes on the course, I thought to myself that I was really going to rip this one hard. As often happens, throwing harder messes with technique. Although counterintuitive, in order to throw further it is usually more effective to be smoother and slower rather than harder and faster. Ignoring this good advice, I threw harder anyway and tripped ineptly on my follow through.

As I did this, I felt my right knee buckle slightly, and it took all my effort not to fall down. The knee hurt a lot. I was unable to play the rest of the round effectively, and was forced to limp pathetically through the back nine. Even more embarrassing, I lost my temper at my own clumsiness and cursed in front of my friend Pete's two-year-old daughter. She comes along for the round and sits on his shoulders patiently playing with her own disc and coming down every few minutes when it is her daddy's turn to throw. Although Pete reassured me that his daughter was paying me no attention and hadn't heard a thing, my dumb throwing decision resonated strongly with the guilt I felt from yelling obscenities in earshot of his little girl.

When my leg gave out three months earlier, just a few days after the original injury, there was no pain and no lingering effects. This time there was plenty of pain and it did not go away quickly. The damage from this mishap was mostly on the outside of my knee, that is, the right side of my right knee. I contacted my doctor who now suggested I get an MRI to check on the inner workings of my knee. I started to think that perhaps something bad had happened after all on Great Misery Island. This sounded like the trailer of a cheap horror movie, and I couldn't help laugh out loud.

An X-ray is useful in confirming that the main bones of the knee are where they are supposed to be, and that nothing is cracked, misaligned, displaced, or broken. It can also reveal fluid and soft tissue swelling, but an X-ray does not reveal structural details of ligaments, tendons, menisci, and muscles. If I had torn or stretched a tendon, ligament, or a meniscus, an X-ray would miss it, but any abnormality would show up clearly on an MRI.

I don't like to waste time and resources on unnecessary tests and procedures, so before scheduling the MRI, I visited dozens of sites online to try to determine whether the MRI was really indicated. My pain was on the outside of my right knee, so I figured that I had either torn the lateral meniscus or stretched the LCL. I learned that both these injuries heal effectively without intervention, but just to be safe nonetheless, I scheduled the MRI for three weeks later, pretty sure that I was just wasting everyone's time and money.

I limped badly for a few days but could still hike and had good strength in the leg. I even took a short family hiking trip to the Berkshires and managed fine. The pain soon began to subside and after two or three weeks the pain completely disappeared. I was sure I had been correct about its cause (a strained LCL, or torn lateral meniscus), but I followed through with the MRI anyway, curious to see what the results look like.

An MRI is an interesting experience. First of all, because of the monster-sized magnets that make the machine function, you must remove all metal or magnetic objects from your pockets, and leave them in a provided locker. A friend of mine once ruined all of his credit cards by accidentally leaving his wallet in his pants, while he underwent an MRI. I was very careful to avoid this.

Once you are metal and magnet free, you lie down inside a long tube, about the size of small coffin, open on both ends. They offered me headphones and music but I declined, expecting to use this time as an opportunity to nap. Some people get very claustrophobic about the experience of an MRI, but I liked it – very soothing and meditative – until the noise began. It sounds like someone banging the outside of the half pipe over and over again with a sledgehammer at irregular intervals. Now I know why they offered me the headphones. They also give you a little button to press so you can tell them if you are freaked out. I eventually got used to the noise, and although I was unable to fall asleep, it was all over in less than a half hour, long before I needed to press the button. They told me that I would receive a copy of the images and the report, and that they would also send a copy directly to the doctor.

When I received the MRI the next day, I immediately threw the DVD into my computer to view its contents. It turns out that an MRI is not a single image, or even a single set of images, but a collection of sets of images, each set taken from a different angle. Indeed, a single set of these images reminds me of a topographic map, where a set of contour lines shows slices of the terrain taken horizontally to the ground. I am familiar with reading "topo" maps on hiking trips, and I am comfortable using the slices to summon up a three-dimensional image of the surrounding mountain and regions.

A major difference between reading an MRI and a topo map is that with a topo map, you don't see the *inside* of the mountain, only the edges. In an MRI, each slice shows the edges and a complete image of what is surrounded by the edges. Also, there isn't just one set of horizontal slices taken parallel to the ground, but many sets of slices each taken at a different angle with respect to my knee. A trained radiologist can look at the various sets and the images in each set, and mentally reconstruct a three-dimensional image of the knee.

I enjoyed looking through the images but I did not have the slightest idea of how to interpret what I saw. What I could conjure from these sets of images had no connection at all to a realistic 3D image. It reminded me of trying to see the image of a bear while staring up at Ursa Major and the Big Dipper. It brought to mind a room of people hopelessly crossing their eyes at the stereoscopic Magic Eye images. "There it is," – if you say so.

Perhaps it is no surprise that it takes quite a bit of practice, training, and experience to read an MRI. Nonetheless, I am proficient at reading English, and as I looked further through the DVD's pages, I found the following report:

MRI OF THE RIGHT KNEE:

TECHNIQUE: Sagittal T1, sagittal, coronal and axial proton density with fat saturation, proton density coronal fat images were obtained.

FINDINGS: The quadriceps and patellar tendons are intact. The anterior cruciate ligament is torn. There is a focal area of increased signal intensity in the posterior horn medial meniscus, which appears contiguous with the inferior articulating surface compatible with a posterior horn medial meniscal tear.

CONCLUSION: TORN ANTERIOR CRUCIATE LIGAMENT. POSTERIOR HORN MEDIAL

The report clearly concluded (in CAPS nonetheless) that I had a torn ACL, and a torn medial meniscus. The posterior horn means the back third of the medial meniscus – the most common place for it to tear. Once again, I had been completely wrong. There were no injuries to my LCL or lateral meniscus; in fact, it was my ACL and medial meniscus that were torn. Indeed, Dr. Berkson explained to me later that although lateral meniscus tears are the most common collateral injury accompanying *initial* tears of the ACL, once an ACL is torn and the knee is unstable, medial meniscus tears are more prevalent when the knee gives out again. This reinforced the notion that I had indeed torn the ACL months earlier in the original hiking accident.

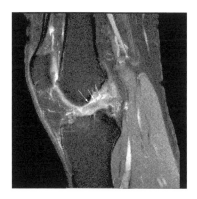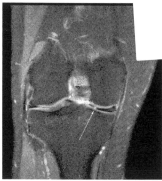

The left MRI image illustrates a side view of the knee with white arrows pointing to the torn ACL. The right image shows a frontal projection with a white arrow pointing to a gap in the medial meniscus.

After I read this report, my self-delusion kicked into high gear. The report was crystal clear, but almost nothing I had learned about an ACL tear matched my experience. I had heard that an ACL tear is excruciatingly painful, and that the pain lasts a long time with great swelling. I had read that most athletes do not walk away from an ACL tear, but get carried off the field. I was told that I would likely hear an audible "pop" at the moment of the tear. Furthermore, I read that if you did not have these experiences, then you most surely did not tear your ACL.

I had fallen and hurt my knee, but stood up and walked it off. I danced at a wedding a few days later – the raucous circle-style dancing of Jewish and Greek weddings, guaranteed to stress any ACL. My original pain and swelling disappeared mostly within a week, and completely after two or three months. My pain from the most recent injury was already gone. Indeed, my knee felt 100%. I heard a slight popping sound at the time of the accident but nothing so different from the normal clicks and snaps that one hears when a knee stretches, twists, or hyperextends. Despite the report, I still did not believe that I had a torn ACL.

It is interesting, but perhaps not so surprising, that normally intelligent people will believe the most unlikely things if they have good enough motivation. You get the idea if you ever heard someone misinterpret a carelessly worded conclusion to a date: "I think he/she really likes me – he/she promised to call sometime." My desire *not* to have a serious knee injury greatly exceeded this kind of wishful thinking - I *really* did not want to have a torn ACL. Rather than accept the facts and reinterpret the last three months in terms of an ACL tear, I clung to the improbable notion that my MRI was switched with someone else's, or that was it was misread.

I may be a stubborn, hopeful, and self-deluded fool but after a while I started to reconsider and had second thoughts like "Why me? Oh crap. Not *my* ACL!" Eventually, sanity kept pressing in and I made an appointment to see Dr. Eric Berkson, an orthopedic surgeon who works with the Boston Red Sox. I figured that anyone good enough for a professional athlete is better than what I needed. Also, two friends of mine, both physicians, and one a sports medicine expert, recommended Dr. Berkson. Indeed, the daughter of one of these friends had torn her ACL playing soccer and had been treated successfully by Dr. Berkson. I felt I was in good hands.

Meanwhile, I had a disc golf tournament the Sunday before my appointment. I decided to test the knee once more before my appointment, thinking that if anything went wrong, I would be seeing the doctor anyway. I played a good round, shooting two under par, putting me in the top five of my amateur division. It was a very respectable showing and I had no pain or episodes of knee buckling, or any other maladies. I thought again that maybe the MRI was mistaken. The next week I joined two buddies on a hiking trip to Mount Moosilaukee in New Hampshire. My knee felt fine – no pain, no instability, no buckling.

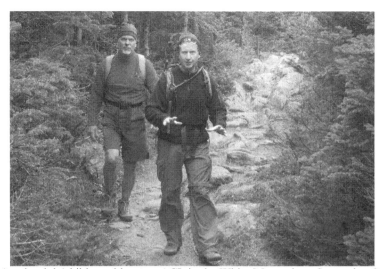

Simonson (on the right) hiking without an ACL in the White Mountains - September 2011

I rode my bike to the appointment. The doctor's office is in Patriot's Place, a very large shopping mall in Foxboro, MA, that doubles as the stadium and home of the NFL's New England Patriots. To save time because I was running late, I took a shortcut around the back of Patriot Place where the deliveries are made, hung my bike over the top of a chain-link fence, scrambled over the fence, and grabbed my bicycle to continue cycling on the other side. A burly angry security guard with a big dog caught me and made me climb right back, bike and all, forcing me to hurry even faster as I rode an extra three miles all the way around. I was in no pain, had no trouble hopping over a fence with my bike, and certainly felt no need for a doctor.

Arriving just in time, I ran up the stairs to the doctor's office, checked in with the receptionist and waited only about five minutes before a nurse called my name. The waiting room was filled with people on crutches, in wheelchairs, wearing braces, grimacing, limping, and in various degrees of pain. Why was I here?

I filled out a large number of forms including personal information, insurance information, medical history, and a short questionnaire.

What is your pain level right now on 0-10?   0

Do you have any persistent pain now? No.

Has your pain increased or decreased in the last two weeks? Uh… No pain.

What brings you here? They say I have a torn ACL.

Do you have any other complaints? I feel fine.

I answered simply and honestly; I felt ridiculous for making this appointment. The people here really needed help and I did not. The vast majority parked their cars in the handicap spots out in front. Well, actually, there is free valet parking for patients, so mostly they walked or were wheeled from the revolving entrance door to the elevator.

The nurse led me to an empty room, set up my MRI on the computer, and told me that Dr. Berkson would be in to see me in a few minutes. As I waited for him to knock on the door, I played around with various plastic models of the knee displayed around the room. I tried to locate the ACL, and determine just what an ACL-deficient knee is like. When I finished exploring the models, I moved over to the computer and scrolled through the MRI images, as I had done at home on my own computer. The images were completely inscrutable. I learned very soon that, among a host of misinterpretations, I had reversed the meaning of black and white. Where I thought I saw a ligament was actually a tear, and where I thought I saw a possible tear there was a ligament.

Dr. Berkson was patient with my questions and assured me without any doubt that my ACL was completely torn. There was no mistake about it. In fact, the ACL was completely missing on the MRI. He could see no remnant or even a stub. He was surprised enough by this to ask if I had ever had any knee injury in the past, thinking logically that perhaps I had injured this ACL years ago but never knew it.

I informed him that my knees had never given me any problems before Great Misery Island. Indeed, I never had even minor knee pain before that, nor had I incurred a leg injury besides a broken fibula 25 years earlier as a result of sliding badly into 3rd base. He shrugged and said that the three months of cycling since the original injury could have "cleaned" away the remnants of a tear originating on Great Misery Island, and that an MRI does not show everything anyway.

Dr. Berkson spent a few minutes examining my knee and confirming diagnostically what he had seen on the MRI. There are a number of diagnostic tests to confirm a torn ACL. The modern "bread and butter" diagnostic for testing a torn ACL is the Lachman test. The test measures the degree of looseness of the tibia relative to the femur. One of the jobs of an ACL is to ensure that the tibia does not move too far forward relative to the femur. A trained clinician can feel the degree of looseness, especially the side-to-side differences between the good leg and the bad leg. A second test, the Pivot-shift, tests the rotational stability of the ACL and can be difficult to elicit in the office. When this test is positive, it virtually confirms the diagnosis. The combination of these tests can be very accurate, sometimes obviating the need for an MRI (except to look for other damage in the knee).

We talked for a while. It turns out he studied computer science before he turned to orthopedic surgery. I am a computer science professor, so we spent a few minutes talking about a subject I actually knew something about. He seemed very bright and confident – traits I admired that put me at ease. Dr. Berkson soon changed the topic back to my knee.

He explained that the way I was presenting was typical, and that it is a myth that *every* ACL injury is a devastatingly painful – carried off on a stretcher – incident. It is possible, if not common, for a person to tear his/her ACL and not know it. Indeed, after a few days of rest and rehab, some athletes return to their sports after an ACL injury never sensing anything is wrong. And, after a few months, their knees will feel 100%; they have no pain and no complaints.

This was sounding good to me. It seemed like I was one of the lucky ones who tear their ACLs and heal without any intervention. "Well, it was nice meeting you – I hope I did not waste your time," I thought to myself.

Dr. Berkson continued to explain patiently that although a very small number of people can ignore a torn ACL, most active people could not return to normal sports without surgery. A fast twist or strong torque will eventually cause their knees to "give out." When a knee gives out, it means the femur moves one way and the tibia moves the other, effectively separating the leg and causing immediate collapse. It is difficult to remain standing when these two bones do not line up on top of each other. And, keeping them lined up is the job of the ACL.

Dr. Berkson explained that instability of the knee, due to the absence of an ACL, eventually results in new injuries with collateral damage to menisci and other ligaments. Besides the immediate effects of these new injuries, the repeated damage to cartilage (menisci) in the knee may bring on early arthritis.

It was about at this point in our conversation that I remembered falling while throwing a disc a few days after the Great Misery Island injury. I also recalled the painful stumble a few months later from an overthrown disc that left me limping for the rest of the round and the subsequent two weeks. It all fit the picture – cycling and hiking caused no instability, and even circle dancing left my knee intact, but the sharp accelerating twisting needed in disc golf was enough to cause knee buckling. My knee had "given out" twice in the three months following my ACL tear: once a few days afterwards, and once three months later. I was lucky the first time, but the second time it surely did fresh damage to whatever menisci and ligaments that had healed.

So what were my options? With a fresh injury, there would be need for rest, ice, and then physical therapy to strengthen the knee before possible surgery. However, my injury was old, and I had already rehabbed the knee on my own, so the options were simply surgery or no surgery.

With a complete tear and signs of instability, the only way to prevent further damage without surgery is to avoid all twisting sports. If I were willing to spend the rest of my life doing things in a straight line, Dr. Berkson would not recommend surgery. I could still cycle, run, swim, but no basketball, disc golf, Ultimate, or skiing. That was a lot to give up.

I asked if I could avoid the instability by being careful and overprotective, but he shook his head. Although my knee had only given way twice in three months, he explained that it was now more likely to give out again. Furthermore, I might get caught up in the excitement of the game and thereby forget to be "careful." Or worse, the knee would surprise me and give out when I was not anticipating any danger.

Dr. Berkson explained to me that just 20 to 30 years ago, ACL replacement surgery was rarely recommended for "older" people, meaning age 35 and up. In those days, the risks were greater, the percentage of success less, and the methods more invasive. If a person could get along fine without having to make sharp side-to-side pivoting moves, then why subject them to risks? Certainly, there are plenty of sports where the action is not primarily side-to-side, including running, cycling, swimming, and even hiking. Someone past their athletic prime could simply avoid "cutting" sports.

Nowadays, it isn't how old the patient is, but how active he/she is. Dr. Berkson was confident that I could not maintain my current lifestyle without repeated episodes of instability. I was not so sure. He was basing his opinion on hundreds of patients, experience, and statistics, while I was basing mine on wishful thinking and my aversion to surgery.

He explained that the standard surgical options nowadays have converged to three reliable methods with excellent outcomes. All of the techniques use human tissue to completely replace the torn ACL, either by *autograft* or *allograft*. An autograft means tissue from the patient, and an allograft means tissue from a cadaver. "Allograft" sounds sexier than "tissue from a dead guy."

Repairing, rather than replacing, an ACL is ineffective. Stitching an ACL back together results in ACL that is not strong enough to avoid a subsequent rupture. And, replacing an ACL with an artificial one, whether made from plastic, rubber, Teflon, silk, polypropylene, or anything else, does not have the appropriate combination of strength, elasticity, and robustness as human tissue.

1. The Patellar Tendon Autograft. This is the "gold standard" and is recommended for younger athletes or professional athletes who need to return to sports quickly with close to 100% performance. The downside is a more painful recovery and a harder rehab program. Also, some patients report lingering pain with lunging or kneeling. Derrick Rose, Tom Brady, Wes Welker and Jerry Rice all had patellar tendon grafts.

2. A Hamstring Tendon Autograft. This has the downside of leaving a very slight but permanent weakness in the hamstring muscle, and the upside of a slightly easier recovery. The outcomes are not so different from a patellar graft, and most athletes return to their sport effectively. Kaya Turski had two hamstring grafts. Hamstring grafts are sometimes necessary in younger patients who are still growing.

3. An Allograft –(tissue from a cadaver). This option allows a much less painful and speedier recovery but comes with a tiny risk of infection from foreign tissue, and a secondary risk of possible stretching, weakness, or failure of the graft.

It is important to note, that after a year, all three methods have similar success rates. That is, if you make it through the rehab program with no issues, then 96% of the time the new ACL, in all three cases, is usually good enough to last a lifetime. Indeed, the chances of injuring it again are no worse than the chances of injuring it to begin with.

Dr. Berkson explained that for or an older person like me (I was 53 at the time), an allograft is the most common recommendation. After all, I don't really need to get *back* to 100%, because at my age I was never 100% to begin with before surgery. However, he said that he was willing to go with either option 1 or 3 for me, depending on what I wanted.

I thanked him for his patience and excellent explanations, and told him I would think about the pros and cons of surgery. I remarked aloud that 6 to 9 months of rehab over the larger time scheme of my life would, in the end, seem insignificant. Dr. Berkson nodded sagely. Meanwhile, he suggested that I get fitted for a sports knee brace. In the interim, or perhaps even over the long term, the brace might protect me from instability, but at the least it would serve to remind me to be careful. I agreed and promised to get back to him. As I was leaving, I asked him one more question: "I just want to make sure I understand *your* recommendation before I go. Do *you* think I should have surgery?"

"Definitely," he answered.

I wasn't so sure. I was instinctively against surgery. By nature, I am averse to any sort of medical intervention. I don't regularly take any drugs. I prefer to suffer through pain for the "feedback" rather than take pain medication. With pain, at least I know what my body is trying to tell me, so I can react intelligently. Artificially reducing pain makes me feel out of touch; and even aspirin and ibuprofen are drugs I use infrequently.

Of course, there are times when the right drug can literally be a lifesaver, and certainly many surgeries are justified and even necessary. The important thing is not whether you prefer intervention or not, but that you take an active role in the management of your health. Every medical decision you make should involve an intelligent discussion with your doctor. The decision of whether to have ACL-replacement surgery is no exception.

My compulsion to ask questions is annoying to some professionals, but I have found that a good doctor, who understands the reasons for common practice, is happy for the opportunity to educate and to share their hard-earned knowledge with a curious newbie. I would even go further. If you insist on understanding the reasons for something, and a professional reacts defensively or answers in an intimidating way, then you should go to someone else for treatment or advice. It may be true that some things are difficult to explain and even harder to understand, but after all, it is your ass on the line, and it is their job to guide and help you. Even ideas that take years to learn can be presented with some clarity at a naïve and elementary level.

For example, I was at first reluctant to undergo the recommended colonoscopy for people who reach age 50. Were the risks worth the benefits? The proctologist I visited was patient and intelligent as he answered my questions. Nowadays there are millions of these screenings done every year, keeping proctologists very busy. It is somewhat controversial whether these screenings are helpful, but it has become the norm for a few important reasons:

- Colorectal cancer is a killer.
- The cancer usually presents itself after age 50.
- Early detection can mean the difference between life and death.

There is also almost no risk in a colonoscopy; the downsides are mostly economic issues: time and money. The only real "danger," is if the doctor messes up badly and punctures the wall of the colon or large intestine with the scope. The chances of this are very slim, especially with a competent practitioner. Nonetheless, when given the option, I elected to undergo the procedure without anesthesia, figuring that if I were awake, a good scream would keep an errant poke of the scope under control. If I were drugged or asleep, and the doctor had a bad day, he would never know for sure if he was hitting a tight curve or pushing his tube through my organs and out my belly button.

I was glad I underwent the colonoscopy. It was fast, uneventful, and the "negative" results were reassuring. Moreover, without anesthesia, I got to ask loads of questions in real-time while watching the video. I really appreciated the biology lesson, and my doctor also seemed to enjoy our conversation. Also, because I declined the anesthesia, I was allowed to drive myself home from the hospital, which for legal reasons is not permitted for patients who have undergone sedation. This was fortunate for me, since I had not lined anybody up for a ride home.

A good friend of mine, when he turned 50, would have nothing to do with a colonoscopy. He is still quite healthy, but seems to prefer being surprised by a cancerous polyp than to undergo the procedure. He is a mathematician by profession and an expert in statistics, so clearly logic is not the only issue at hand. Emotions can transcend the numbers. I think most people have a fear of a "plumber" snaking an eight-foot tube through their large intestine. And, assuming you can overcome that fear, there is still the unpleasant "preparation." This involves emptying yourself completely through strong laxatives and a liquid diet for 24 hours. Fear and discomfort notwithstanding, for the most part, it is irrational to object to a colonoscopy screening.

On the other hand, there are many good reasons to object to surgery. Surgery has real risks. Although ACL replacement is routine compared to other surgeries, and it is far more advanced and reliable than it was just 20 years ago, the overall *a-priori* success rate is still no better than 95%. That means there is at least a 5% chance I could get worse, and in so many different ways: permanent stiffness or pain, graft failure or tear, infection, persistent instability, temporary or permanent numbness, etc. Not to mention the teeny chance that the anesthesia alone might kill me.

Why should I take a perfectly fine knee and subject it to these risks just so I could continue participating in twisting sports for the next 20 years and avoid occasional instability? I decided that I would test the knee over the next half a year and see how it faired through my normal activities. If I had no more episodes of instability, then I would reject surgery, and remember to wear my brace whenever I participated in a sport like skiing that severely stresses the ACL.

Reinforcing this line of thought was a conversation with a cycling friend, Jordan, a pediatrician a few years older than me, who had unknowingly torn his ACL as a young man. Jordan finally learned of his injury when he experienced some meniscus pain after completing a marathon years after his ACL tear. A colleague took a scope to his knee to look around and found that there was no ACL. Jordan insists that in all his active life he never had an unstable episode with that knee. When I asked him to what he attributes his good fortune, he said "quads." He does have strong quads, but perhaps more relevant is that his main sports are running, cycling, and sailing. He does not regularly play basketball, soccer, tennis, or any other twisting sports. There was no way to know if I could repeat his excellent record but at least I was encouraged.

I continued playing disc golf and doing my normal 20-mile roundtrip commute to work by bike. Since the two original knee-buckling disc-throwing episodes, my body learned to protect itself – my knee had not buckled in months of hard throws. I started to believe that the combination of my strong cycling quads, good luck, and self-protection might keep me stable forever. I noted to myself that I had not engaged in any basketball pickup games or in any sport requiring hard pivoting, so I planned one last test.

At the end of every semester, I organize an Ultimate (Frisbee) game with my college students. That would be the final test. I would play normally and if everything went as expected, I would leave the option of surgery on the table.

In December 2011, six months after my injury on Misery Island, and three months after I first learned of my torn ACL, I scheduled the game. I decided not to wear my brace, because

a. I was pretty sure I did not need it,

b. I wanted this test to finally confirm without any doubt that my knee was stable, and

c. I hated the feel of the brace anyway.

As I always do, I spent my time trying to involve all the students and making each one feel like he/she was contributing and having fun. The game is competitive but filled with good sportsmanship and spirit. I felt great. I am not as quick as I used to be, but I can still play "handler" very well. The handler in Ultimate is like the point guard in basketball. He/she greases the offense, makes passes, organizes the cutters, but very rarely cuts or dives to catch a pass. It's a good role for a middle-aged guy quite a bit slower than he once was.

The Ultimate game had been going on for about 15 minutes when I picked up the disc about midfield, and my student Brendan on the opposing team played up close to defend against my throw. Out of the corner of my eye, I noticed one my teammates sprinting toward the end zone a couple of steps ahead of her defender. There were a number of cutters close by looking for a short pass or "dump."

I moved my right foot pivoting on my anchored left foot and faked a backhand short pass to a teammate who was well covered. I quickly shifted to my forehand stance, pivoting again on my fixed left leg, simultaneously cocking my hips and wrist back. Planting my right leg hard around Brendan's left side, I accelerated my hips forward counterclockwise, followed by my right shoulder and right wrist, delivering a clean flick under his left arm. I hoped that the disc would be caught in the end zone, but I never saw what happened to that pass.

The moment I rotated my hips forward, my femur moved right past my tibia sending me to the ground in pain. My students quickly gathered around me, and the next thing I remember was looking up into a sea of concerned faces. Brendan looked guilty, and the rest of the students seemed nervous, wondering whether their professor was just clumsy or having a heart attack. Embarrassed, I stood up, reassured Brendan that he defended properly, and confirmed that I was okay. I tried to run a few steps but I was unable to continue playing without a lot of pain. It was not the way I hoped to end the day's play. My students were as kind as could be, but I felt like I had somehow let them down. As I limped back toward my office and watched my students walking off the field, I had a vision of my denial and self-delusion marching hand-in-hand out of my brain like two angry teenagers sheepishly storming out of the house. "Good game," I told everyone.

I rode my bike home and mumbled to my wife Andrea that my knee had given out, and I had some pain on the inside (the medial meniscus area). She, of course, had recommended that I wear my brace, and I was not very convincing when trying to explain to her why I had not worn it. I don't know whether or not the brace would have actually protected my knee, but the upside of not having worn the brace is that at least I learned definitively that the knee was unstable. Andrea could tell I was at a moment of crisis.

I did a quick calculation assuming my knee gave out every two to three months for the rest of my active life. Five times a year for 25 years made 125 injuries. That would collectively be at least a year of pain and recovery, not to mention long-term damage and early onset of arthritis. Was surgery worth it to avoid this scenario? I knew the answer. My knee failed the test. With the reality of my unstable knee etched in my brain, I knew that surgery was the next step.

The pain from this failed test lasted six weeks, much longer than the pain from the original torn ACL, and twice as long as the re-injury three months later. I made a doctor's appointment as soon as possible so that I would not change my mind as the pain started to subside. Dr. Berkson was not surprised to see me. He listened to the whole story, reconfirmed the instability of my knee with the Lachman test, and massaged the medial meniscus on the inside of my knee, which hurt.

We discussed the options for surgery, which for me were limited to a patellar tendon graft or an allograft (a cadaver's tendon). The patellar tendon graft would give better long term outcomes and a higher chance to be 100% active again, while being more painful and requiring a harder rehab. It also would allow me to get off crutches sooner – perhaps even as soon as a couple of days after surgery. The allograft would have some minor risks of infection, might not heal as strongly or effectively as a patellar graft, would require me to be on crutches for six weeks to protect the graft, but would be far less painful. I opted quickly for the patellar tendon option because I wanted to get back on my feet as soon as possible. I asked Dr. Berkson whether he had any strong opinion, and he reassured me that my preference was fine.

We then discussed the rehabilitation. I was clueless about the extent and nature of the rehab despite all the reading I had done. I had no sense at all of how badly this surgery was going to set me back. I asked Dr. Berkson if I could be back teaching at the college after a week. He said maybe two weeks, but if I could sit while lecturing then I might be able to go back after one week, depending on whether I was still on crutches and how I was recovering. I asked how soon I could get back to commuting by bike. He smiled and said that after two weeks, I could start on a stationary bike, more for range of motion than for exercise, and work my way up to a strong effort when I had full range of motion. He said that for safety concerns, real cycling should wait for at least two to three months.

Whoa! I did not anticipate being off the bike for that long. I was clearly in over my head here. This was far more sacrifice than I expected, and I still did not appreciate the extent of it. I was not used to this kind of setback; maybe nobody is.

We scheduled the surgery for the Friday before my college's Spring break. This would give me ten days of rest and rehab before I would have to be back at work, and give Dr. Berkson a chance to return from his duties at Red Sox spring training camp. I finished the appointment by signing many sheets of paper stating that I understood the procedure that was being proposed, that I knew the risks, and that I was willing and able to do the necessary exercise and work for successful rehabilitation.

During the next three months leading up to surgery, I second-guessed the decision many times especially after the pain from my torn meniscus subsided. However, I was signed up, committed, and was not going to change my mind. I would undergo ACL replacement surgery nine months after my scrambling accident that caused the tear.

Modern ACL surgery is quite different from what it was 40 years ago, and even 20 years ago. Today's surgery is more precise and less invasive because it is done arthroscopically. The surgeon cleans, drills, and measures with very cleverly designed tools, through small holes in the skin. The arthroscopic technique minimizes the trauma to the knee during surgery and is a great improvement over the techniques of the past - where the knee was splayed wide open to facilitate the procedure.

My surgery was one of a few options, but it represents a typical procedure.

The basic surgical ACL replacement consist of two parts:

a. Harvesting and preparing the new ACL.

b. Attaching the new ACL.

There is also the matter of cleaning up collateral damage to menisci and other structures, which are caused by either the original injury or by subsequent injuries due to the leg giving out. This means anything from a repair of a meniscus, tendon, or ligament, to a trimming or removal of loose or torn meniscus pieces. The extent of this extra work depends on the severity and type of the injury, so there is no standard.

The details of acquiring and preparing the new ACL vary depending on the source of the new ACL. Using a patient's own tissue is thought to provide the greatest chance for a complete and long-term return to full performance and function, but this advantage comes with a price. The surgical removal of a section of tendon requires a long recovery and rehabilitation to regain strength and function. With dead tissue from a cadaver, only the site of the ACL replacement itself needs to heal properly. Because there is no second site of trauma, healing is quicker and less painful, there is less post-operative muscle atrophy, and surgery is faster and simpler. Using cadaver tissue is a good choice for patients with collateral damage to other parts of their knee, where minimizing secondary sources of pain and weakness is an important concern.

The second part of the surgery is more challenging. The attachment of the new ACL is complex business and demands skill, patience, and resourcefulness. The remnants of the old ACL must be removed and the site for the new ACL cleaned and prepared. The area is flushed with water continuously to keep the view clear, and there is very little bleeding. Holes must be drilled into the femur and tibia to receive the new ACL, and these holes must be lined up just right so that the new ACL will not be pinched when the knee is bent, and so that the new ACL twists appropriately when the knee is extended.

You can watch a live surgery on YouTube, with one doctor doing running commentary while he carries on a dialogue with another who is performing the surgery[14]. It is fascinating to watch even if you are squeamish. It's carpentry without spare parts.

The most important part of the surgery is matching the normal attachments of the new ACL to their original locations on the bones of the femur and tibia. This placement of the new ACL is by far the hardest part of the surgery and where mistakes can be made. I heard a story from one physical therapist that sounded to me like an exaggeration, but regardless of its accuracy, the story underscores the possible errors that can occur during surgery. While watching an ACL replacement surgery during training, he reported seeing a surgeon mangle part of an

[14] https://www.youtube.com/watch?v=8P-RPG8hT90

autograft replacement as it was screwed into the femur tunnel. The surgeon carefully backtracked to evaluate the situation, examined the damaged replacement tissue, shook his head in frustration and embarrassment, lost his temper, and threw his stool across the operating room. He quickly regained his composure and completed the surgery using an emergency allograft that was available for this purpose.

The knowledge of how and where to place the new ACL is much improved today compared with the past. After affixing the replacement ACL, the surgeon tests the strength and placement of the new ACL by watching its movement as he bends the knee. When the surgeon is satisfied with placement and alignment of the new graft, he/she closes up all holes and incisions. With the replacement tissue in hand, a skilled surgeon can replace an ACL carefully and safely in one to two hours. The time needed for a complete surgery with an autograft can take an hour or more longer because of the necessary harvesting.

ACL surgeries are usually performed with the patient under *general anesthesia* – where the patient is rendered completely unconscious. Without general anesthesia, surgery would be horribly painful, and practically impossible for all but the most pressing needs. General anesthesia is a bit mysterious but very safe and reliable. Although we know much more about it today than we did 50 years ago, there is still plenty we do not know about exactly what happens to someone when they are "put out." With full anesthesia, a patient has no muscle control, and the brain seems to shut down in certain ways. No pain is felt, no memories are retained, and even breathing needs to be regulated. The anesthesiologist vigilantly monitors heart rate, blood pressure, EKG patterns, pulse rate, respiration, and even your level of consciousness. Some patients spontaneously breathe themselves, some need the help of a ventilator, and some need help sometimes but not other times. Nowadays, with a combination of science and intuition, an anesthesiologist routinely, and with complete control, brings a patient to the brink of death, effectively allowing him/her to safely undergo otherwise unbearably painful procedures. Soon after the procedure is complete, the anesthesiologist brings the patient back to life. It is an amazing part of modern medicine.

General anesthesia is not without risks. Since all gagging and coughing is suppressed, it is important the patient has an empty stomach to prevent inadvertent choking or inhalation of fluids or other particles. This is why you are ordered not to eat the day before surgery. A less serious risk is that some people feel nauseous after recovering from general anesthesia. Overall today, a healthy person will almost always tolerate general anesthesia well, with risks of death or serious problems lower than 1 in 100,000.

The standard practice today for ACL replacement surgery is to supplement general anesthesia with a femoral nerve block on the affected leg. A nerve block is a type of *local* anesthesia – where only a certain area of the body is rendered numb to prevent pain. The femoral nerve is one of the two major nerves serving the leg. The other is the sciatic nerve so familiar to people suffering from bad backs. Generally, the femoral nerve serves the front of the leg and the sciatic nerve serves the back of the leg. The nerve block on the femoral nerve is primarily for pain management subsequent to surgery.

I had a talk with the anesthesiologist about whether I had to undergo the nerve block. I explained that I preferred a little pain along with the accompanying helpful feedback than to have a numb useless leg. He carefully explained that without the nerve block, he would have to pump me with more painkillers during surgery, which would increase my grogginess, delay my waking, and raise my risk of post-surgery nausea. Furthermore, the numbness would only last 24 to 48 hours, and would help me avoid taking painkiller medication later on. He convinced me to do the nerve block.

I persisted with my anesthesiologist, and asked him a question that he probably did not expect. If he was numbing my leg, did I then really need general anesthesia? After all, if the leg was numb I would be immune from any pain, so why undergo the risks and heavy-handedness of full anesthesia?

My anesthesiologist wasn't sure I was serious but after he realized that I was indeed dead serious, he was kind enough to give me a carefully thought out and convincing answer. He explained that with only the femoral nerve blocked, it was very likely that I would feel pain at some point in the two-to-three hour-long surgery. The pain might come as the drill got close to the back of my leg, or perhaps because I moved or jumped at the wrong time. In any case, even if I could tolerate the pain in short doses, I might not emotionally be able to tolerate it for the length of the procedure, and putting me under in the middle of the procedure was no easy task.

He anticipated my next question, and before I could ask, he added that he couldn't/wouldn't do an additional nerve block on my sciatic nerve, to completely deaden the leg and allow surgery without general anesthesia. He explained that when I woke up, my leg would effectively be like a piece of driftwood connected to my body at the hip. It would be disorienting at the least and dangerous at the worst. In any case, general anesthesia was the standard thing to do, and he recommended no variation. I thought I could see the anesthesiologist roll his eyes as he left my bedside. I could hear him thinking "No anesthesia? What a nut!"

Nonetheless, I desperately wanted to be awake during the surgery so that I could follow what was going on and ask questions. The whole procedure fascinated me; I was amazed by the intricate plans of carpentry with my bones and ligaments taking the place of wood and screws.

On the other hand, the surgical team just as desperately wanted me to fall asleep so they could do their jobs without having to answer my questions, or worry about me screaming in pain or freaking out from the sound of a drill and the smell of bone powder. I think that if I had persisted with even one more question, the anesthesiologist would have put me out on the spot.

Dr. Berkson came to in to see me, double-checked which leg was injured, and marked his initials on the appropriate leg. It is not unheard of for a distracted surgeon to operate on the wrong leg, arm, or even kidney. Routine safeguards are automatic. Indeed, surgeons are trained never to pass the ACL replacement from person to person, and instead to wrap it automatically around his/her finger before moving it from one place to another. Dropping the ACL replacement graft on the floor would necessitate a time-consuming special cleansing procedure; and in the worst-case scenario, it might require the disposal of the graft, and the need for an emergency allograft.

The anesthesiologist then gave me a shot in the leg to relax me, followed by the nerve block. I said goodbye to my wife, and was wheeled into the operating room. No general anesthesia had yet been administered, and I remember being nervous that I wouldn't fall asleep right away. I talked to Dr. Berkson and the rest of the surgical team for about 30 seconds, at which point the drugs were released into my body, and the next thing I remember, I was awake, shaking my head, and looking up at my wife again. I do not remember anything during the two and ½-hour long surgery; I do not even remember dreaming. I had left home at 6:30 AM, and I was back at home by 2:30 PM that same day: two hours waiting and prep, two hours or so of surgery, two hours of post-surgery recovery, and a half-hour travel each way.

The physician's report appears below. It describes the diagnosis, findings, and surgical procedure. Basically, the ACL replacement went smoothly. Unfortunately, the injury to the

76

inside of my right knee sustained in the Ultimate game was serious. My medial meniscus was so badly ripped up that it could not be repaired; Dr. Berkson needed to cut a small section of it clean away. The missing meniscus is nothing that I notice now or will likely notice in the near future, but it will almost surely affect my knee 10 to 20 years down the road. Because there is less padding there than there used to be, after years of heavy use it is likely that early arthritis will set in. For this, I have no one to blame but myself. If I had not waited so long to schedule the surgery, and hadn't tested the knee over and over again for six months after the initial injury, I almost surely would have been left with my menisci intact.

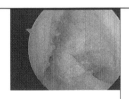 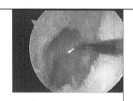 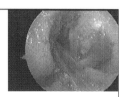

These images from arthroscopic surgery demonstrate:

Left: A torn ACL,
Center: A newly created tunnel at the start of the ACL in the femur, and
Right: The final graft in position in the two tunnels in the knee.

Surgery was over but the long road of rehab had just begun. That's another story.

Chapter 4 – Questions and Answers: A Quick Reference

"It is better to know some of the questions than all of the answers."

James Thurber, author

This informative chapter is organized using a question/answer format. It is the first place to look for quick and accurate information about the basics of ACL injury and surgical repair. The questions are ordered logically, each one leading to a natural follow up question, so that a first reading of the chapter can be accomplished smoothly from start to finish.   Alternatively, feel free to skip from question to question, depending on your interests, and come back to the details on a subsequent read.   An already educated, oriented, and focused reader can treat the chapter as a frequently asked questions (FAQ) reference section.

There are many things about ACL tears and replacements that are well understood, supported through various studies, and universally accepted by surgeons. A number of ideas and practices, although based on solid scientific logic, are a matter of opinion and style. Finally, a few isolated myths persist among the public and even among some surgeons, despite no conclusive evidence.   The questions and answers in this chapter will help you distinguish between these categories.

What is the ACL?

The ACL is an abbreviation for the anterior cruciate ligament, one of four major ligaments that together hold your knee in place. Together with the posterior cruciate ligament (PCL), the two ligaments cross over each other in the center of the knee connecting the femur (your thigh bone) to the tibia (the larger lower leg bone), and providing stability when your knee twists, turns, or cuts. The other two ligaments, the lateral and medial collateral ligaments (LCL and MCL), provide connectivity on the sides of your knee. The LCL connects the femur to the fibula, the smaller lower leg bone that sits on the outside of your leg, and the MCL connects your femur to the tibia.

Are there are other structures in the knee?

The knee is a complex joint with ligaments, tendons, menisci, bursae, bones, nerves, muscles, and blood vessels. Together these structures provide strength, stability, and cushioning, which allow a great variety of pain-free activity and motion. Of these structures, the menisci are very important. The C-shaped pieces of cartilage are located in between the bones and act as shock absorbers, protecting a second type of cartilage — the articular cartilage — that coats the ends of the bone. Loss of the articular cartilage is called arthritis. The loss of menisci directly results in earlier onset of arthritis.

How is an ACL injured?

An ACL is a pinky-sized piece of tissue connecting your femur to your tibia. When an ACL is stretched too far and too fast it can rip apart just like a rubber band or flexible rope. Normally, an ACL is strong enough to handle at least 1725 Newtons (about 450 pounds) of force[15], so day-to-day activities will not cause it any distress. However, there are all sorts of different ways to exceed 450 pounds of force. Most ACL injuries occur without an external agent. That is, the athlete simultaneously jumps and twists, or lands and pivots in a violent way. Although virtually all athletes weigh far less

---

[15] http://emedicine.medscape.com/article/89442-overview

79

than 450 pounds, it is possible to magnify the force of one's body weight by acceleration and leverage. A sharp change in direction, with an anchored pivot point can do it.

Although many ACL tears occur without an external force, some ACL injuries occur as a result of a "hit." Typical would be a collision in football or soccer. A 250-pound lineman tackling you on a dead run, and clipping your knee from the side, is plenty of force to tear an ACL.[16]

What does an ACL injury feel like?

A variety of experiences are reported. Everyone falls down and suffers some level of pain. Some hear a "pop." Some get up on their own, some with assistance, and some need to be carried away. There is often, but not always, swelling, and the degree of swelling varies. Pain and swelling last a minimum of two to three days and as much as two to three weeks. Many athletes are pain-free and 100% functional within a few weeks; indeed, some are not even aware that they have torn anything. Unfortunately, the great majority of people with torn ACLs experience episodes of instability, or even knee buckling, when they go back to their sports. Instability leads to not trusting your knee to support you during sharp twists and maneuvers. This affects performance and can cause unnatural motion and secondary injuries.

Can I continue an active life with a torn ACL?

---

[16] A Comparison of Autogenous Patellar Tendon and Hamstring Tendon Grafts for Anterior Cruciate Ligament Reconstruction Ryan M. Dopirak, MD; Damon C. Adamany, MD; Robert N. Steensen, MD Orthopedics August 2004 - Volume 27, Issue 8

Very few people manage to tear their ACLs and avoid instability. An unstable knee can give out under stress and cause a person to fall, collapse, and sustain new injuries. There are testimonials from people who avoid instability, but many of these people self-selected subsequent activities that did not stress their ACLs. If all you want to do is ride a bicycle and run in a straight line, then you may never notice your torn ACL. However, any turning, sharp starts and stops, and/or jumps may cause your knee to buckle. More commonly, a person with an unrepaired but asymptomatic ACL tear presents ten years later with degenerative arthritis, presumably due to repeated and excessive wear and tear on knee cartilage. Although functionally stable, the knee is not functioning normally internally and the patient is unaware of the ongoing, slow, and debilitative cartilage damage. Thus, even if you find that your knee is stable, over time you still might require some sort of surgical repair.

Is an ACL tear often accompanied by other ligament or cartilage damage?

It is possible to injure just your ACL with no damage, or only minor damage, to other tissue; however, it is common for an ACL tear to be accompanied by other injuries. Both the MCL and LCL can be torn, and the medial and lateral menisci can be damaged. A common combination, known as the unhappy triad, is a torn ACL, MCL, and medial meniscus. This happens often in football when a knee is hit hard on the outside. It is much less common to tear the PCL, in part because it is much thicker and stronger than the ACL, and in part because the kind of injury that stresses the PCL is different and less common from the cutting/planting/twisting motion that tears an ACL. The time needed

81

for full recovery from ACL replacement surgery far exceeds the time needed for the MCL, LCL, PCL, or various menisci to heal.

How is an ACL tear diagnosed?

There are two major clinical tests for testing for ACL tears: the Lachman test and the Pivot-Shift test. An MRI may confirm the diagnosis.

What is the Lachman test?

The most reliable way to test for an ACL tear in the physician's office is the Lachman test. The patient is lying down on his/her back and relaxed. With the leg flexed slightly at about 20 to 30 degrees the doctor stabilizes and supports the upper thigh near the knee, simultaneously pulling the lower leg forward with the other hand. The thigh is pressed downward towards the table, while the lower leg is lifted upwards. This painless diagnostic test effectively attempts to measure how far the tibia can move forward relative to the femur. Normally the tibia moves only about 3 mm, but with a torn ACL a physician can feel a movement of up to 10 to 12 mm.

The medical books have a more technical description. *Distal femur* means the part of the thigh closest to the knee; and *proximal tibia* means the lower leg close to the knee. An *anterior translation force* means to pull forward.

"One hand secures and stabilizes the distal femur while the other firmly grasps the proximal tibia. A gentle anterior translation force is applied to the proximal tibia. The examiner assesses for a firm/solid or soft endpoint."[17]

---

[17] http://www.sportsdoc.umn.edu/clinical_folder/knee_folder/knee_exam/lachmans.htm

The Lachman test is difficult to do correctly, but a positive test is very reliable. False negatives are possible because a damaged leg can still exhibit plenty of stiffness due to muscle spasms or strong supporting muscles. A good reading depends on the expertise and experience of the surgeon or practitioner. A trained clinician can feel the degree of looseness along with the firmness of the endpoint. It isn't so much the absolute looseness that matters as much as the difference in looseness between the good leg and the bad leg. Comparisons between the laxity in the good and bad legs is one way to improve the reliability of the test. It takes skill and experience to perform this test and evaluate the results effectively. Trying this yourself at home is unlikely to be informative or helpful.

What is the Pivot-Shift test?

This test is harder to perform in the office than the Lachman test and more difficult to describe. Basically, the physician attempts to twist the leg, push the knee inward, and allow the tibia to move out of place and back into place. If the ACL is torn, this position causes the knee to "pop" indicating a positive pivot. Due to muscle guarding, an injured leg can resist or dampen the popping motion, making the test less reliable in the office than the Lachman test.

Dr. Berkson and his student attempted this test in both of my preoperative appointments, but each time the test was inconclusive (false negative) due to muscle guarding. The pivot-shift test is used more commonly and more successfully before surgery when the patient is under anesthesia and does not resist. In this context, it serves as a final confirmation of the knee's instability and supporting evidence of a likely ACL tear. Indeed, Dr. Berkson performed the test with positive results after anesthesia was administered, just prior to my surgery.

Once again, the medical description is more precise and intimidating. *Valgus* means outward away from the body, and abducted means away from the axis of the limb. Think bowlegged. An axial load is pressure on the front of the knee joint.

With the hip flexed about 20 degrees, and abducted slightly, the tibia is externally rotated while a valgus stress is placed on the knee. With a strong axial load, the knee is flexed from full extension to about 20 degrees. If the ACL is not functioning, the tibia will shift back into place at about 20 degrees of flexion causing a popping sensation.

Like the Lachman test, it takes practice to be able to administer the pivot-shift test accurately and it requires experience to evaluate the results. These are not meant to be do-it-yourself tests.

Are there non-clinical tests to confirm an ACL tear?

The standard non-clinical test is the MRI. An MRI is magnetic imaging, so it is painless, uses no harmful radiation, but is expensive and can be noisy. MRIs give a series of cross-sectional images that a trained radiologist or surgeon can interpret and thereby construct a mental three-dimensional image of the internal workings of the knee. However, there is a big difference between interpreting an MRI and examining the knee internally with a scope. Most of the time, a surgeon cannot know *exactly* what damage has occurred until he/she looks directly inside the knee.

Is an MRI necessary after or before a clinical examination to diagnose a torn ACL?

An ACL tear is fairly well-indicated by the tests performed by the surgeon in the office. Therefore, most physicians do not rely on MRIs for diagnosing a torn ACL if clinical tests seem indicative and reliable. An MRI can confirm a tear suggested by a Lachman test, may be able to help distinguish between a complete tear and a partial tear, and can assess other damage to the knee. However, an MRI is expensive and it may not be cost effective to order it. In many cases, with or without an MRI, the surgeon will not know the complete extent of the injury until he/she is able to see it with his/her own eyes during surgery.

Can an ACL partially tear?

Most ACL injuries are complete tears, but a partial tear is possible. Unfortunately, distinguishing between a complete tear and a partial tear is not as clear as it might seem, and looking at the MRI is not enough. The ACL tends to stretch before it tears. For this reason, the ACL may seem intact on the MRI, but in actuality is not functioning well enough to protect the knee. An ACL that produces a positive "pop" on examination in the operating room (a positive pivot-shift test) is not functioning and needs to be replaced. This is considered a complete "tear" of the ACL even though the ligament still looks intact.

A partial tear of the ACL is the case where the ACL shows some sign of injury on the MRI, yet the pivot-shift test remains normal. In this case, the ACL can still protect the knee and has not stretched "too much." Because the pivot shift test needs to be done in the operating room to be most effective, it sometimes requires an examination in the operating room to declare an ACL injury a partial tear. The good news is that if the pivot-shift test is normal, the ACL should be expected to gradually improve over time and get better without surgery.

It is difficult to get accurate figures on what percentage of tears are complete because not all partial tears are reported and even complete tears go undiagnosed. Some studies suggest that only 10% of ACL injuries are partial tears, but this is difficult to confirm.

Do I need surgery for a partially torn ACL?

While a completely torn ACL cannot reconnect, a partial tear has a chance to repair itself. Remember, a partial tear of the ACL is a stretch injury to the ligament that still allows the ligament to function. This ligament remains at risk for further injury if it is stressed too early. If the ligament heals, then surgery is unnecessary. If the partial tear provides enough stability, then after a suitable rest period, an athlete may return to active sports without surgery. In these cases, it is usually a good idea to wear a knee brace for extra protection and as a reminder to be careful until the ligament heals back to full strength.

Can a brace protect an ACL or a healing ACL?

This is a controversial topic. Most clinicians believe that a high-end, well-fitting sports brace can add some additional stability to the knee and protect the ACL ligament to some extent. This may be especially true for direct contact injuries. A brace alone though, is not enough to replace a non-functioning ACL and the knee can give out while wearing a brace, causing further injury to the knee. An ACL brace cannot substitute for surgery or a complete muscular rehabilitation and recovery.

Is it true that women athletes tear their ACLs more often than males?

This is a commonly heard piece of wisdom that is not exactly true but is also not quite a myth. Indeed, it is men that tear their ACLs more often than woman, but this statistic includes contact injuries, like being tackled in football. An estimated 30% of ACL tears are contact injuries, and the vast majority of these are men. For *non-contact* tears, however, it is more common to see women tear their ACLs.

There are many theories as to why women suffer more non-contact ACL tears than men, but nobody really knows for sure. One theory is that the "tunnel" in which the ACL sits is narrower in woman than in men. This narrowness causes a *guillotine effect* in which the ACL is pinched during a severe and tight twist. Others believe that the predominance of non-contact ACL tears for women may be due to their lower quadriceps strength, weaker balance (neuromuscular control), and/or different styles of landing from a jump based on anatomical differences. Other theories include the effects of estrogen on ligament properties. It is likely that all of these play some role in this increased prevalence of injury. Importantly, addressing strength, balance, and neuromuscular control in general can reduce risks of future ACL injuries.

Is there any way to prevent ACL injuries from happening in the first place?

There are many coaches and trainers that implement preventative programs and training meant to minimize the chances of an ACL tear. These prevention programs are becoming more popular as ACL injuries become more common. These programs are especially prominent in women's high school athletics, because it is well established that proportionally, teenage female athletes tear their ACLs more often than any other group. Preventative strengthening and neuromuscular control exercises are a popular approach because the best way to "treat" an ACL injury is to avoid suffering one in the first place. These preventative measures are the "seatbelts" of athletic programs all over the US. For example, the Mass General Sports Performance Center in Foxboro, MA focuses on prevention as much as it does on rehab.

Are all ACL tears related to sports and athletics?

Not all, but most. Anyone can tear an ACL at any time merely by stumbling or tripping. And, a traumatic injury, like a car accident, can cause ACL tears. In this scenario, an ACL tear is almost certainly accompanied by other non-knee injuries.

Can a torn ACL be repaired?

It took years of experimenting and studies to learn that repairing an ACL does not work. The repaired ligament either fails again quickly, or does not function like the original. The only viable surgical option today is the replacement of the ligament. There are a few people around the United States studying new technologies to repair a ligament including giving specific growth factors to the ligament. Unfortunately, these are still in the early testing phases, and have not yet been shown to work in humans.

Can an ACL be replaced with an artificial ACL or other non-human tissue?

Artificial replacements, both synthetic and from animals, were attempted decades ago and found to be ineffective over the long term. There have been some modern attempts to reintroduce synthetic grafts using a hybrid approach. A more detailed discussion of synthetic ACL replacements and their use in state of the art modern treatments can be found in Chapter 7, along with the history of ACL surgery.

What are the options today for treating a torn ACL?

The main option used today to treat a torn ACL is surgical replacement using human tissue. The other option for treating a torn ACL is non-surgical - simply leave the ligament torn and rehabilitate the knee. Since the ACL does not grow back or reattach spontaneously, this conservative option implies that a person will attempt to function normally without an ACL. Thus, the athlete must stick to sports and activities that avoid lateral acceleration, pivoting, and cutting.

When is surgery for a torn ACL *not* recommended?

Assuming that a patient is either young or wants to return to active life, surgery is usually indicated. The option of avoiding surgery is feasible only when the knee shows no signs of instability, and/or the patient is willing to avoid high-demand twisting sports. Otherwise, the dangers of recurrent injury to menisci and resulting long-term progressive arthritis, call for surgery.

Examples where surgery is not recommended include:

- A partial tear with no signs of instability.

- A complete tear with no signs of instability during low-demand sports such as running, swimming, or cycling, along with a willingness to give up high-demand twisting sports, such as basketball, soccer, skiing, or tennis.

- A sedentary lifestyle, with a willingness to forgo any sports activity.

Most athletes who have a hope of returning to their sports opt for surgery. There are stories of athletes avoiding surgery and managing successfully over the long term without an ACL; however, that is the rare exception rather than the rule. A much more common scenario is when an athlete incurs additional injuries and damage to cartilage due to knee instability by attempting to return to sports without surgery. Such people often wish they had undergone surgery immediately.

What about a young child with a torn ACL?

It is more and more common for a growing child to tear his/her ACL. Additional consideration for the growth plates around the knee must be given to prevent growth disturbances. While previous recommendations were to delay surgery until the child is almost fully grown, specialized techniques to reconstruct the ACL avoiding these growth plates have resulted in better results for younger kids. This is a specialized procedure requiring specialized training.

What are the options for surgical replacement?

Surgical replacement uses either an autograft or an allograft. An autograft is tissue from the patient, and an allograft is tissue from a cadaver.

What exactly is an allograft?

An allograft is dead tissue that is cleaned, washed, irradiated, and then frozen. It can be taken from a variety of sources including a patellar tendon, hamstring tendon, Achilles tendon, and various other tissues. Because the allograft tissue is dead and processed so thoroughly, it contains almost no protein antigen, and therefore poses no risk of rejection by the immune system of the host. From the point of view of the immune system, the body treats an allograft very much like a synthetic replacement.

Why don't we use fresh donor tissue for ACL replacements?

Fresh donor tissue from a parent or other willing person is not used for ACL replacements because of the high chances that the graft will be rejected. Making sure of a good tissue match is expensive and inconvenient when alternative more economic methods are just as effective. Finally, a processed allograft can be tested for infection and is thereby generally safer.

Does the choice of autograft versus allograft affect surgical success rate?

The success of an ACL replacement over the long term is dependent primarily on the skill and experience of the surgeon, rather than on the choice of graft. The rate of complete success is around 90%. Nonetheless, each graft does have its own unique set of risks/rewards.

Recent research has shown that allografts have a very high failure rate in those patients less than 20 years of age. Cadaver allografts tend to stretch out more than autografts in this younger population. Interestingly, in an older population (older than about 40 years of age), allografts may be a better choice, avoiding some complications of surgery.

What is the main advantage of an allograft?

The big advantage of an allograft is less pain during recovery. There is no harvesting of tissue with an allograft, and so there is no second site of trauma to heal. There should be a good reason to wreck otherwise healthy tissue, and an allograft avoids this. Ironically, this advantage is also a risk. Less pain earlier in the recovery period, combined with a potentially weaker graft, makes it more likely for a patient to push himself/herself too hard and too early, thereby injuring the graft.

What is the main downside of an allograft?

An allograft is not as strong as either the patellar or hamstring autograft, because an allograft is dead tissue and it is treated to kill infection and prevent disease. Due to this, many researchers suspect that an allograft will weaken, stretch, or fail, faster and more readily than an autograft, thereby decreasing its useful life.

Over a period of 10 years most studies show no difference in outcomes and strength between allografts and autografts[18]. Use of an allograft in older patients may prevent complications including pain in the front of the knee. This, and the less painful and easier recovery, is one reason that an allograft is a common recommendation for older patients.

Although no long-term studies have conclusively confirmed the weakness and earlier failure of allografts in comparison with autografts, some studies have shown a

---

[18] http://www.orthoassociates.com/SP11B35/

higher failure rate of allografts among younger patients, possibly because of the greater stress they put on the ligament.[19] For this reason, an allograft is rarely an option offered to a young and otherwise healthy athlete. The exception to this is when a young patient presents with multiple ligament injuries, in which case, minimizing extra trauma becomes a concern.

Are there any other risks or downsides associated with allografts?

Another disadvantage of an allograft is that hard recovery is delayed because the patient remains on crutches for up to six weeks after surgery. This conservative recovery is necessary because it is important to protect the dead tissue of an allograft until it grows strong enough to handle more stress.

An extremely rare risk of an allograft is the transmission of a serious disease such as HIV or hepatitis. The problem is that any treatment (typically radiation) strong enough to kill all disease in an allograft with certainty is also strong enough to alter the tensile strength of the tissue. Therefore, to keep the allograft strong for the years ahead, allograft tissue is never guaranteed to be 100% free of disease. Nonetheless, the risk of transmitting disease is extremely small; in particular, the chances of transmitting HIV through an allograft are around one in a million.   These risks are minimized by testing each graft "to the best of science's ability" and by using bone banks which are non-profit.

One might guess that an allograft carries a risk of rejection, but that is not the case. Interestingly, autoimmune rejection of an allograft is rarely an issue because there

---

[19] http://www.orthoassociates.com/SP11B35/

is very little protein antigen in the graft. The graft is composed mostly of collagen, which from the immune system's perspective is relatively inert, like metal.

What is the main advantage of an autograft?

The advantage of an autograft is that it gives the best chance for a complete 100% return to pre-injury performance. An autograft is more likely than an allograft to thrive quickly when relocated. Professional athletes planning to return to their sports almost always opt for an autograft. Autografts remain the gold standard and avoid problems of cadaver tissue, including likelihood of stretching out and viral infection.

What is the main downside of an autograft?

The main downside of an autograft is a harder initial recovery. The harvesting of the graft causes damage to the area where the graft was taken. The affected tendons, muscles, and/or ligaments need lots of time to recover.

Patellar tendon autografts may increase the chance of having pain in the front of the knee when kneeling. This risk is highest in those who have pre-existing arthritis under the kneecap and is lower risk in younger individuals.

Hamstring autografts may be associated with a larger infection rate, and may carry some risk of hamstring weakness in rehabilitation and in future sports. While scientific studies have not yet demonstrated any specific weakness from harvesting the hamstring tendons, recent studies suggest that that harvesting the hamstrings may affect some patients more than others.[20]

---

[20] https://www.ncbi.nlm.nih.gov/pubmed/28205075

Can a graft get infected?

Note that both allografts and autografts have similar risks of bacterial infections - around one in a 100. Treatment with antibiotics usually works, but sometimes the infection does not respond to antibiotics, and the graft may need to be replaced. In extremely rare circumstances, a bacterial infection of the graft could cause death.[21] Most of the time, an infection means additional surgery to wash out the knee and possible revision surgery in the future. Intravenous antibiotics are often required in these settings.

Which is more expensive, an allograft or an autograft?

In all cases, allografts are expensive in comparison to autografts. There is a cost involved in harvesting, processing, and storing cadaver tissue.

What happens to the graft after it is put into place in the knee?

When the replacement graft is secured in position in the knee, it undergoes a process called *ligamentization*.[22] [23] This fancy word means that the tissue needs to get used to life as a ligament. This transformation takes place over a period of many months, during which time the tissue develops the strength of the original ACL and exhibits similar functionality.

A great deal of this process involves the establishment of a strong blood supply - revascularization. Also, nerve connections need to rewire in order to improve

---

[21] http://www.orthoassociates.com/SP11B35/

[22] The "Ligamentization" Process in Human Anterior Cruciate Ligament Reconstruction With Autogenous Patellar and Hamstring Tendons, A Biochemical Study, Keishi Marumo, MD, Mitsuru Saito, MD, Tsuneo Yamagishi, MD, Katsuyuki Fujii, MD, *Am J Sports Medicine, August 2005, vol. 33, no. 8, 1166-1173*

[23] The "Ligamentization" Process in Anterior Cruciate Ligament Reconstruction: What Happens to the Human Graft? A Systematic Review of the Literature, *Am J Sports Med November 1, 2011 39 2476-2483*

proprioception – that important sense of our own body's position, balance, and strength.[24] This revascularization and rewiring occur more quickly, and probably more completely, with autografts than with allografts. Generally, surgeons allow weight bearing on an autograft earlier than on an allograft, but recommendations vary greatly.

How does ligamentization affect the care of your knee after surgery?

Due to the ligamentization process, one must be more careful not to damage a graft in the early weeks after surgery. Avoiding a tear of the graft in the newly operated knee is paramount. If the new graft tears, the patient needs to wait months for the trauma of the failed surgery to dissipate, and repeated surgery does not usually have as good of an outcome. Therefore, regardless of the type of graft, most surgeons are very conservative regarding the care of the knee for the first six weeks after surgery.

Indeed, an autograft gets *weaker* for the first six weeks after surgery before revascularization kicks in effectively and strength starts to increase. In effect, the old live tendon tissue dies, and reincarnates as a ligament. Therefore, during the first six weeks after surgery, many surgeons recommend wearing a full leg brace, which is much larger and more restrictive than a sports brace. Not only is this the time when the graft is weakest, but it is also the time when the patient is most likely to fall due to the effects of surgery. The brace also serves as a reminder to be careful and as extra support in case of a fall. You have surely seen post-surgery patients hobbling around in the full brace. Photos of the full brace and the sports brace appear in Chapter 5.

---

[24] Arthroscopy. 2003 Jan;19(1):2-12.Proprioception of the knee before and after anterior cruciate ligament reconstruction.

Some surgeons also recommend crutches during this period, while others allow weight bearing as soon as the patient can tolerate it. Regardless of your doctor's specific management of your care after surgery, generally, all doctors are more conservative with an allograft compared to an autograft, since an allograft starts as dead radiated tissue.

What are the options for allograft tissue?

Allografts are taken from the same tissue used for autografts – i.e., the patellar tendon or hamstring tendon, as well as other tissues including the tibialis anterior tendon - the tendon at the bottom of the large muscle that runs on the outside front of the shin, and the Achilles tendon in back of the heel. There is a wider choice for an allograft because there is no fear that the loss of the tissue will impact the donor. Some surgeons prefer one kind of tissue to another, believing, for example, that in the long term, a hamstring tendon may stretch and weaken less than a tibialis anterior tendon. However, no long-term studies have confirmed the benefits of one allograft type over another.

Interestingly, ACL tissue itself is not used for allografts for three reasons:

1. It is difficult to harvest the ACL without damaging it, and even harder to capture the bone endpoints, a technique necessary for a strong replacement. If a surgeon were to willy-nilly cleanly extract the ACL with the bone endpoints from a cadaver, the process would likely render other parts of the knee unusable for other replacements and procedures.

2. Sizing the ACL is very important, and it would be difficult and time consuming to find a cadaver whose ACL matched the patient's ACL. With other tissues, the sizing is more flexible and easier to manage.

3. In practice, the patellar, hamstring, Achilles, and tibialis anterior tendon allografts all have good track records, so there is no reason to prefer a real ACL for replacement.

Thus, using ACL tissue to replace an ACL is not necessary to ensure a good outcome. Indeed, using ACL tissue for an ACL allograft replacement would be more difficult and possibly less effective than using other tissues.

What are the options for autograft tissue?

An autograft is usually taken from the injured leg in order to preserve full functionality in at least one leg. The primary choices for an ACL autograft are:

- Patellar tendon (middle third)
- Hamstring tendon
- Quadriceps tendon (less common)

Does it matter which autograft option is used?

Most studies show that in the long term, each choice is equally effective and strong. The patellar tendon graft is still thought of as the "gold-standard," but with new techniques for hamstring harvesting, most studies do not show a significant difference in function between the two. Today the hamstring graft is a quadruple bundle of four strands constructed from two hamstring tendons. After a few months of healing, this bundle is much stronger than the original ACL. The patellar tendon graft also ends up stronger than the original ACL after six months of healing, but is not quite as strong as the hamstring. Either way, when positioned properly and healed completely, either replacement graft is strong enough to allow a full return to sports for a lifetime.

Do surgeons specialize in a particular kind of autograft replacement?

Some surgeons tend to use more of one kind of autograft than another. Experience is crucial, and the techniques for harvesting and placement of the various autografts are different. Your surgeon is likely to recommend a particular kind of autograft based on his own expertise, and on your age, temperament, motivation, and level of fitness. The more important factor for successful ACL replacement is a surgeon's skill in harvesting and placement of the autograft, rather than the kind of autograft that is chosen.

How is the patellar tendon graft harvested and affixed in place?

With a patellar tendon graft, the surgeon cuts away the vertical middle third of the tendon along with a two small fragments of bone at each end, one from the patella (kneecap) at the top end, and one from the tibia at the bottom end. The two outer thirds of the patellar tendon, each of which remains connected to the patella on top and the tibia on the bottom, are sewn together laterally to close the gap left by the removed middle third. A video by Dr. Bertram Zarins at Mass General Hospital [25] gives an excellent animation.

The harvesting of the patellar tendon leaves the natural connection of tendon to bone intact at both ends of the tendon. The harvested tissue graft is about the same size as the original ACL, about 1 cm by 10 cm, with small fragments of bone on each end. The surgeon drills small tunnels in the femur and tibia, and threads the replacement tissue

---

[25] https://www.youtube.com/watch?v=q96M0jRqn7k

into place where the old ACL used to be. With implantable screws, he/she affixes the bone at one endpoint of the graft into the femur tunnel and the bone from the other endpoint into the tibia tunnel. The patellar bone fragment and femur join strongly together over time, as do the tibia bone fragment and tibia.

What are the specific advantages and disadvantages of the patellar tendon graft?

The most significant advantage of the patellar tendon replacement is the potential for a complete return to full performance. The bone-to-bone anchoring of the patellar tendon autograft creates a strong new ACL that heals fast and reliably, and integrates quickly into place. Also, since the patellar tendon is almost the same size as the ACL, small placement adjustments are relatively easy to perform.

The main disadvantage of a patellar tendon graft is the slightly more painful initial recovery, because the patellar tendon is severely, but temporarily, weakened. Overall recovery times are unchanged. However, pushing too hard too soon can result in a patellar tendon tear, so the rehabbing athlete must balance patience with hard work.

Another disadvantage of the patellar graft is that the removal of a piece of patella can leave the patella fragile. This can cause a patellar fracture, particularly when an athlete tries to return too quickly to his/her sport. Jerry Rice, the hall of fame wide receiver, fractured his patella in this exact circumstance. A good surgeon carefully replaces the piece of bone removed from the patella with small pieces from the tibia, so that the bone grows back into place readily, leaving the patella more robust.

Other disadvantages of a patellar replacement include:

- temporary or permanent pain in the knee, especially when kneeling on the affected kneecap,

- greater chances to experience minor loss of extension in the joint, and

- risk of chronic patellar tendinitis even after months of rehabilitation, especially if the athlete pushes too hard.

And finally, after a patellar tendon replacement there is almost always some minor numbness that persists below the kneecap. The extent of this numbness diminishes in size and intensity over time, but in some cases, permanent numbness may persist.

How is a hamstring autograft harvested and affixed in place?

With a hamstring tendon, two tendons are removed from the hamstring muscles in the back of the thigh, and four strands are bundled together to create the new ACL. An important distinction between the hamstring graft and the patellar graft is that the hamstring graft does not have bone at the ends. In this case, the surgeon needs to affix the tendon directly to the femur and tibia tunnels. This is done with a variety of clever techniques often including a metal button that sits just outside the bone. Other techniques are possible.

What are the specific advantages and disadvantages of the hamstring graft?

One disadvantage of the hamstring graft is that the bone-to-tissue connection requires a longer period of time before the hamstring tendon attaches effectively into its new location. Moreover, this healing time is less predictable than the bone-to-bone patellar graft. Thus to minimize the danger that the hamstring graft shifts location, some physicians recommend using crutches longer and delaying weight bearing in the first six weeks after surgery. Finally, the longer, less predictable healing time for hamstring grafts may change rehabilitation processes at the end portions of recovery.

On the positive side, a quadruple-strand hamstring graft is stronger than the patellar tendon graft (at least in the lab). This advantage, however, is not as important as it might seem because when fully integrated and healed, both autografts are stronger than the original ACL.

A more significant advantage of the hamstring graft is that there is less potential for long-term pain in the knee. Also, recovery of the quadriceps muscle is faster after surgery because the patellar tendon remains intact.

The most significant disadvantage of the hamstring autograft is that the hamstring in the harvested leg sometimes exhibits mild long-term (or permanent) weakness relative to the hamstring in the non-harvested leg. This is less common than it used to be because of improvements in harvesting technique; nonetheless, a very serious athlete might be more likely to choose the patellar tendon autograft. Normal folks will generally not notice the difference in hamstring strength after careful rehab.

Does it matter if an autograft is harvested from the damaged leg or the healthy leg?

Most surgeons harvest the replacement graft from the same leg that was injured. This avoids affecting the "healthy" knee and allows focus on only one knee during recovery. Interestingly, those in favor of harvesting a graft from the uninjured knee report that the more difficult initial recovery (because both legs are recovering) protects the ACL surgery. Sometimes, due to repeated or multiple injuries, there is no choice; only one leg might be available. The ultimate decision depends on your particular case and should be discussed with your surgeon and physical therapist.

Would a synthetic or artificial graft be better than a natural graft?

Undoubtedly, a successful synthetic graft would be a great breakthrough. A synthetic graft has no risks of infection. A synthetic graft shares the allograft's advantage of no secondary harvest site trauma. There are no secondary risks of long-term weakness at the harvest site. The surgeon opens up the package and in it goes. The recovery time is quicker and the risks less.

Yes, an effective synthetic graft would be wonderful; however, all attempts so far have met the same fate. Whether Gore-Tex, Dacron, carbon fiber, or polypropylene, synthetic grafts eventually wear out, fray, and spread little particles through the joint and the lymph system. Typically, the knee becomes perpetually swollen and eventually the graft must be removed and replaced.

One day, medicine may finally succeed at finding a viable synthetic graft and the days of autografts and allografts will seem antiquated and primitive. In the meantime, future research in this area includes a hybrid of synthetic and natural grafts. Hybrids of synthetic material and allografts have been attempted successfully, and more advanced hybrids are being considered. Using synthetic material as scaffolding, scientists are trying to implant and grow a patient's own ligament cells around the scaffolding, thereby creating a new ACL with the exact characteristics of the original. The success of this strategy needs to be tested.

What does arthroscopic surgery mean?

Arthroscopic surgery means that the surgery is done through small holes using scopes to see what is going on. All ACL replacements today are performed arthroscopically. Scars are minimal and trauma to the knee is minimized. Be aware, however, that the harvesting of autografts is not arthroscopic, and that is why allografts are so much less invasive.

Is surgery an urgent option or can I wait safely and think about it?

Most surgeons insist on a healing/rest period of at least one to two months between injury and surgery, so that the knee presents without swelling and other trauma. This has been shown to improve outcomes. As long as you are careful not to reinjure the knee, taking a few weeks to think about your choices is the best advice. The longer you wait, however, the more likely your knee will give out, and the more likely you can injure something else in the knee. It is common to suffer medial meniscus tears and other collateral damage if you continue to aggressively use an ACL-deficient knee. Indeed, I lost part of my medial meniscus because he kept stressing and testing the knee for six months after his initial injury. This has dramatic implications for risks of future arthritis.

How does age affect the decision for surgery?

Generally speaking, anyone with an active lifestyle should consider surgery. Although it was rare 30 years ago to recommend ACL replacement surgery to middle-aged athletes, the good outcomes resulting from modern techniques have made such recommendations commonplace for athletes in their 50s and 60s. As a person gets older, the advantages of an allograft usually outweigh the disadvantages, so that allografts are often the recommended choice.

What should I expect right after surgery?

You will go home the same day of your surgery, and you probably won't feel too good. You will be pumped up with narcotics, painkillers, and a nerve block on your leg. Your leg will look like a watermelon, and you will not recognize the normal contours and shape of your knee. You will need crutches to move around, and you may need to take pain medication to remain comfortable. You will probably not be able to move your bad leg at all for a day or two without the assistance of a CPM machine.

What is a CPM machine and when should I use it?

A CPM (continuous passive motion) machine is a contraption that bends your knee for you as you rest your leg in it. It can be set to various speeds and angles depending on your pain and flexibility. You use the CPM machine as soon as you return home from the hospital for a variable amount of time. Not everyone requires use of a CPM machine. In fact, there has not been any study showing that using it makes a large difference in outcomes. Some surgeons recommend it to preserve motion after surgery, while others use it in special circumstances such as re-growing cartilage. A picture of a CPM can be found in Chapter 5.

How many hours a day should I use the CPM machine?

Some surgeons recommend using it anytime you are lying down, including when you are sleeping. Others may not have you use it at all. In special circumstances, such as treating a cartilage injury in your knee, the CPM may need to be used up to 18 hours a day! You will learn to love your CPM machine, because without it, you could do almost nothing helpful for your knee in the first few days after surgery.

What is the purpose of the CPM machine?

The CPM serves several purposes. One of the most important uses of the CPM is to get your leg to straighten out completely as soon as possible. It is crucial to get your new graft used to complete knee extension as soon after surgery as you can. This prevents permanent limitations in range of motion. Most surgeons would say that getting at least 90 degrees of bending by two weeks after surgery is optimal. The use of a CPM can help this. The CPM can also be important in special circumstances where cartilage is being regrown. In this setting, the motion of the knee nourishes the growing cartilage.

Many surgeons recommend wearing a safety brace whenever you are *not* using the CPM machine. Warning: Do not use wear the brace while using the CPM machine, as the brace can prevent natural bending.

When can I stop using the CPM machine?

Listen to your surgeon about using the CPM machine, as there are many different thoughts about this.

Will there be bandages on my knee?

Your knee will be wrapped in a dressing and probably have a compression sock around the dressing to maintain good blood flow. The holes and/or cuts (incisions) from surgery will have surgical tape on them called Steri-strips.

When can I take off the surgical dressing?

After a couple of days, you can remove the surgical dressing on your knee. However, do not take the surgical tape (Steri-strips) off your wounds until your physician tells you to remove them. The tape is there to keep your skin together while the holes and sutured cuts heal and disappear.

How soon after surgery can I take a shower?

Remember that submerging your knee under water (in a bath or pool) is never recommended until a few weeks after surgery. A shower, however, may be possible earlier. Different surgeons will have different opinions about this and you should ask your surgeon. For most wounds and incisions after surgery keeping them clean and dry is the best practice. If the incisions are small enough, it is often possible to get them wet in a shower at the second day after surgery.

Nonetheless, taking a shower after the first day or two is tough because it is very important not to fall, and trying to balance on one leg in a slippery shower can be tricky. If you fall, you will feel like an imbecile. And, much worse than your feelings, a bad fall could result in you being back on the operating table rather than rehabbing. Many patients opt for a shower chair or other such helpful aid.

Will I be able to use the toilet after surgery?

This will be difficult for the first two to three days. Leaning on crutches, you will need to lower your body weight, supporting yourself on one leg while keeping your bad leg straight out in front of you. If you can suffer the indignity, get a family member to help you sit down; you can remind them to leave when you are all settled.

Can I manage on my own at home without assistance after surgery?

You will definitely need someone to drive you home from surgery. For the first few days, it is preferable to have someone give you some assistance and tender loving care. Certainly, you will benefit practically and psychologically from support for as long as possible. However, after the first week, you should probably be fine on your own if necessary.

What should I do while I am lying around the first week after surgery?

Try to move your leg by doing the simple early exercises recommended by your doctor. If you can't do anything, use the CPM machine and read so that you don't go stir crazy after three hours of up and down. Once you have removed the surgical dressing and gauze compression wrap, it is a good idea to clean the knee, dry it, and keep compression on it for the first week or so.

There are some exercises that you can start after surgery. Moving your ankle up and down can help improve blood flow from the lower legs. Also contracting your thigh muscle (quadriceps) in an exercise called the "quadriceps-set" can help teach the muscle to activate and prevent atrophy.

How often should ice my knee? And what is a Cryo-Cuff?

Ice is one of the best ways to decrease pain and swelling. In general use as much as ice as possible, for at least about 20 minutes at a time. Sometimes, the hospital will provide you with an ice pack that simultaneously ices and compresses the knee. This is sometimes called a Cryo-Cuff (although there are other brand names of similar products); the cuff wraps around your knee with Velcro straps. The Cryo-Cuff comes with a neat system so that you can replace the ice water from an insulated thermos without having to remove the cuff. During the first week or two after surgery, you should ice the knee constantly to get the swelling down. The cuff can be left on when using the CPM machine. A photo of a Cryo-Cuff appears in Chapter 5.

How long until the swelling in my knee subsides?

The immediate and horrible melon-like swelling will disappear after a few days. However, your knee will be warm/hot and large relative to the good knee for at least two to three months. Icing the knee will be a long-term project, and it is important for quicker and more complete healing.

How long will I need pain medication?

This is a very personal matter. Some people do not use any pain medication. Others use prescription medications like oxycodone for the first couple of days/weeks. If you do use the prescription meds, consider taking them in advance in order to "get ahead" of the pain. Waiting until the pain is bad, may leave you with a few hours of suffering until the meds kick in.

When the pain is not severe, an over-the-counter drug like Tylenol and Ibuprofen can also be used to reduce pain and swelling. Remember that taking too much Tylenol (more than the bottle recommends) can be very dangerous. It is rare to need the prescription drugs past two weeks.

What can go wrong after surgery?

The major bad things that can happen once you get home are very rare, but you must watch for them. Firstly, you can get an infection. In that case, your leg will usually become more painful, more swollen, and redder, rather than just the opposite. Secondly, you can get a blood clot, which has similar symptoms. Massaging the leg as soon as you can stand the pain is worthwhile and helpful. If you have a history of blood clots, your surgeon may have you take other medications to thin your blood.

Your surgeon will likely give you a number to call whenever you have any concerns or discomfort. Do not hesitate to call. An untreated infection or an undetected blood clot can have serious consequences, not the least of which is the need for additional surgery.

After the first two weeks, the main thing that can go wrong is injuring the graft by falling or twisting. Follow your doctor's directions and treat the leg very conservatively for at least six weeks.

Should I rub the harvest site if I had a patellar tendon autograft?

After around two weeks, the sutures over the patellar tendon harvest site should be healed, and you can rub the site. Indeed, massaging the site will help break up scar tissue and will help the skin glide smoothly for a more complete recovery. Just make sure not to massage too early or too hard otherwise the skin can come apart, and you will be back at the surgeon's office to reattach it.

Will my leg shrink or atrophy?

It does not take very long to lose muscle mass when you stop using your leg. Most people notice some atrophy and shrinkage, and sometimes it can be significant. The more quickly you begin exercising and rehab, the less atrophy you will experience. In all cases, the leg will grow back to its normal size eventually with physical therapy. Note, that the change in your leg size will affect correct adjustment of a support brace.

Is there anything I can do to prevent my leg from shrinking or atrophying?

One of the reasons the thigh muscle (quadriceps) atrophies is that knee swelling itself tells the quadriceps not to fire. Early physical therapy and beginning quadriceps-setting exercises can keep the quadriceps firing and minimize atrophy.

How long after surgery must I wear a supporting brace?

This depends on your surgeon's recommendations. While some surgeons do not use a brace at all, other surgeons expect you to wear the brace at *all* times for the first six weeks after surgery in order to minimize the risk of injury to the graft. This includes when you sleep. Some doctors recommend *locking* the brace when you sleep, in order to keep your leg fully extended. Other surgeons recommend the brace only when you are moving about. Either way, the brace should *not* be worn while in the CPM machine, because it may impinge on the normal bending movements of the leg, and after the first week or two, the brace not need be worn while sleeping.

How do I adjust the brace?

After surgery, the doctor or physical therapist will help you adjust the brace so that it gives you maximum support and safety while not impinging your normal movement. Refitting the brace is inevitable. You should learn how to adjust the brace yourself if/when your leg atrophies and subsequently strengthens. Be meticulous about refitting when necessary. If the brace slides or loosens, even walking will be difficult. You may be worse off with a badly fitted brace than without one at all.

What if I fall or have an accident after surgery?

Your surgeon's conservative recommendations regarding movement, crutches, and the safety brace, are geared to avoiding an accident in the first six weeks after surgery at all costs. From the surgeon's point of view, outside of a serious infection, the worst thing to happen after surgery is that you fall or have an accident. Damage to the graft or simply moving it out of place will necessitate new surgery. And, the outcomes of a second surgery are generally not as good as the first. If you fall or injure yourself after surgery, contact your surgeon immediately.

How long after surgery until I can go back to work?

This depends on what you do for a living. You can return to a desk job after about one to two weeks. If you need to stand most of the day, then two weeks is the minimum. If you are very active for a living, then you may need a month or more of rehab before you can return to work.

Can I drive after surgery?

If your ACL replacement is in your driving leg, then normally it takes four to six weeks to be able to drive again. You must make sure that in an emergency situation you can safely and effectively hit the brakes with the injured leg without risk of re-injury. If your replacement is on your non-driving leg, then you can drive as soon as you can walk, perhaps in as fast as a few days. If you drive a standard, then get some friends to chauffeur you around for a while.

How long after surgery until I can walk without crutches?

This depends on the kind of graft you had and on the recommendations of your particular surgeon. Generally, with an autograft, you can get rid of the crutches as soon as possible, as early as two days after surgery in the best-case scenario. Keep in mind that "walking" will be labored and abnormal for a couple of weeks, but the faster you start to walk normally without a limp, the better your rehab will go.

How long after surgery until I can run?

If you are asking this, then you are a great candidate for rehab, but you need a dose of reality. Hard running cannot be attempted for at least three months and usually four. First of all, your new graft will not stand the strain of running, and could move before it sets into place. Second of all, running will be very painful and asymmetric. You need to regain your ability to run, pivot, and cut only after your strength, agility, and good form has returned sufficiently.

How long will I be in rehab?

You will be rehabilitating your knee actively and daily for at least nine months. In the beginning, this may be several times a week. In the end, it will be less often. After this, you will be able to exercise normally and will likely be back to your normal sports and exercise program. Your knee and performance will continue to improve for at least two years after surgery. Wes Welker's stats in his first two seasons after surgery confirm this.

How long after surgery until I am able to go back to my sport?

The earliest you can return to your sport is approximately nine months after surgery. If you are a professional athlete rehabbing with a team of therapists, eight hours a day, and seven days a week, you might be able to cut two months off this schedule. Either way, you should expect your knee to feel about 90% to 95% when you first return to your sport.

How long after surgery until I should expect to feel 100 percent?

Even if you return to your sport after just nine months, you will not usually be able to reproduce your pre-injury form until many months later. Even professional athletes notice a slow and steady improvement for two years or more after surgery.

How long after surgery before I start rehab and physical therapy?

You will start exercising at home immediately after surgery, doing very simple exercises such as heel slides and leg lifts. Even these will be difficult soon after surgery. After about two weeks, you will see your surgeon for a post-surgery evaluation, and that is a common time to begin physical therapy twice a week, maybe more often if you are a serious athlete.

How many hours a day, days per week, should I expect to work on rehabilitation?

This depends on your motivation. You should exercise every day. Missing a day once in a while is not a disaster, but should not become a habit. You need consistent effort. Your PT will be thrilled for you to spend up to two hours a day of exercise sets, stretching, and stationary cycling. If you can do more without re-injury, that is better. You can get by with about one hour a day, but you will surely fall behind if you expect to show up and do your work only at the PT meetings.

Does the number of hours per day of rehab change as the months pass by?

As the months go by, you will get stronger and be able to do many more things. The frequency of your PT visits will certainly diminish every few months, from two to three times a week, to once a week, and finally, to once every two or three weeks.

However, for nine months, you must continue to work at least an hour a day to maintain shape and improve your knee's function.

What would be different if I were a professional athlete?

These days, the subspecialty of Orthopaedics Sports Medicine is prominent enough that there are very few differences between the care that a professional receives and the general public. The biggest difference is the oversight that professional athletes have in their recovery process. Team trainers ensure that the rehab process begins immediately and that every step along the way is followed. Professional athletes have time every day to dedicate to their rehab and realize the importance of this part of the equation.

Because of its predictable reliable recovery, professional athletes most often utilize a patellar tendon autograft for their ACL reconstruction.

For those looking for more information or other points of view, there are a number of sites online that the curious and industrious patient can investigate[26] [27] [28] [29] [30] [31]. These sites are not all organized carefully, nor is each particularly comprehensive, but together they provide plenty of content that a critical reader can feast on.

---

[26] http://sportsci.org/encyc/aclinj/aclinj.html
[27] http://www.txsportsmed.com/acl.php
[28] http://www.orthoassociates.com/SP11B35/
[29] http://ismoc.net/knee/patientACL.html#Ch4-
[30] http://www.kneesurgeryacl.com/index.php
[31] http://www.sportsdoc.umn.edu/clinical_folder/knee_folder/knee_exam/lachmans.htm

Chapter 5 – Rehabilitation: Two Steps Forward, One Step Back

"It's just a slow process. You've got to [regain] confidence in your leg. You've got to get confidence in your abilities. You've got to heal mentally and physically. It's just a matter of time."

          Greg Camarillo, Miami Dolphins wide receiver

Most of the injuries we suffer, both small and large, heal relatively quickly and completely. A bruise or scrape from a minor fall is better in a week; a broken limb heals in six. A pulled or torn muscle might require a few months if it is a very serious tear; and torn or stretched tendons take at most a year. Even chronic, debilitating, and painful lower back pain often resolves itself within a year.

In contrast, ACL surgery will set you back a long time. For an average person, the rehab alone for an ACL replacement is a *minimum* of nine months. To reach the point where one cannot distinguish between the injured knee and uninjured knee is more like 2-3 years. It may likely be the longest rehab of your life.

Although the graft itself is almost completely healed after six months, the supporting muscles of the legs, hips, and abdomen need more time to return to their pre-surgery condition. Without proper strength and balance supporting the knee, the new ACL will have much more work to do, and could fail under a heavy stress. A good outcome after nine months has you back to running and normal sports, with swelling and pain mostly gone, and strength close to 100% of pre-injury. Nonetheless, it typically takes an additional year or more before an athlete's performance is back to pre-injury form.

It is not just the body that needs rehabilitation, but also the mind. An athlete needs to learn to rely on a leg that has been unreliable for months. He/she needs to learn to trust the healed knee. Many athletes say that this part of the rehab is the most challenging and frustrating.

Long after the early pain and weakness has disappeared, the mind protects the body from injury by not allowing the athlete to go all out. Patience is required while muscle memory is regained, technique relearned, and confidence rebuilt. Wes Welker was back on the field in less than nine months looking strong, but his return season was, by his standards, a mediocre year of less than 90 receptions. He hit his stride in his second season back, more than 18 months after surgery, leading the league with over 120 receptions. He noticed the difference. And, if he did, then you will too.

Professional athletes, who are exceptional to begin with, who do not have to deal with other jobs and responsibilities, and who benefit from physical therapists and doctors monitoring their progress round the clock, can be back at their sports after 6-7 months, but they are the rare exceptions. Genetics, super effort, and professional support can speed up the process only so much. Time is required to allow the new graft to reach 100% strength, and shortcuts are a recipe for disaster. This is especially true for hard-working athletes who, after four months, may *feel* like their knee is 100%, but the new graft and the damaged patella and patellar tendon may not be ready. Early stresses on a graft that has not yet grown to full strength may loosen or weaken the graft, and early stresses on the patella and surgically altered patellar tendon may result in new injuries there.

Jerry Rice, perhaps the greatest NFL wide receiver of all time, was back on the field less than four months after ACL replacement surgery! He had the "gold standard" patellar tendon replacement, which gives the strongest overall result for getting back to pre-injury performance. Despite doctor's warnings, Rice felt he was ready to return to full contact NFL football after only four months. In his first game back, he cracked the patella from where the graft was harvested.

He was out the rest of the season. Rice eventually made a full recovery, the correct way, patiently working through the rehab program.

Indeed, for the patient, the difficult part of ACL replacement surgery is the nine months of rehabilitation. Successful outcome of surgery is dependent on two things: a competent surgeon, and a diligent patient willing to do the rehab. Without a consistent and steady effort over a long period of time, eventual return to full sports will be delayed, and the possibility of re-injury increased.

The basic plan of ACL rehabilitation is simple: get the knee back to normal and protect the graft while you do. The sooner you get moving and your muscles activated, the faster you will see improvement. However, the key word is patience. Reinjuring the knee or tearing the new graft is a disaster that must be avoided at all costs. A second ACL replacement generally does not go as well as the first.

Here is a general overview of the rehab plan based on my surgeon's notes and the program set up for me by my physical therapists. Recovery is a multiphase progression. Your PT suggestions may vary. Rehab is slightly different for an allograft or hamstring autograft, but overall, your physical therapist will give you a collection of sheets and diagrams illustrating various exercises.

Phase 1 (0-2 weeks)

The goals of this phase are to:

- Protect the reconstruction – avoid falling
- Ensure wound healing
- Attain and maintain full knee extension

- Gain knee flexion (knee bending to 90 degrees)

- Decrease knee and leg swelling

- Promote quadriceps muscle strength

- Avoid blood pooling in the leg veins

- Prevent scar tissue from binding patella – manipulate the patella

- Prevent anterior knee pain

- Start strengthening exercises for quads and hamstrings

The use of a Cryo-Cuff to provide cold compression, and a CPM machine for help with knee bending is ubiquitous throughout this phase.

Some exercises in this early phase include:

- Wall Slides

- Quad tighten

- Quad tighten up and down

- Calf lifts

- Back slides quad thrust

- Towel slides side

- Elastic knee pull

- Step-downs

- CPM Assisted Knee Flexion

- Towel Squeeze - Sit in chair, squeeze rolled towel between knees for 5 seconds. Relax & repeat.

- Calf-Raises

- Walk without crutches

Phase 2 (2-6 weeks)

The goals of this phase are to:

- Protect the reconstruction, avoid falling

- Ensure wound healing

- Maintain full knee extension

- Begin quadriceps muscle strengthening

- Restore knee flexion to at least 90 degrees and ideally up to 130 degrees

- Regain good balance and control

- Reestablish normal gait without crutches

Exercises in this phase have a twofold purpose: balance and strength.

Strength

- Stationery Cycling

- Mini squats

- Step-ups

- Mini Lunges

- Leg Press

- Bridges

- Hip Abduction w/ Theraband

- Hip Extension w/ Theraband

- Chair Scoots

  Balance

- Wobble board
- Stork Stand
- Static Proprioceptive hold/ball throwing

Phase 3 (6-12 weeks)

The goals of this phase are to:

- Protect the reconstruction, avoid falling.
- Maintain full knee extension.
- Attain full knee flexion.
- Walk with normal heel-toe gait with no limp.
- Regain full strength and power by training and conditioning.
- Increase agility and balance.

  Phase 2 exercises continue as needed, and new exercises that can be performed include:

  - Jump & Land drills
  - Hopping and Jumping: forward, backward, sideways, up and down stairs.

Phase 4 (12-16 weeks)

The goals of this phase are to:

- Regain full muscle strength

- Reestablish cardiovascular conditioning

- Begin sports specific training

- Start running

Exercises are running and sport specific.

Phase 5 (16-36 weeks)

The goals of this phase are to:

- Continue running

- Fully return to sports

- Practice cutting, pivoting, and sprinting

- Practice hopping and jumping

- Successfully perform agility tests

The following exercises are used to test the ability of the knee to withstand cutting and planting maneuvers.

- Standing Vertical Jump: Jump straight in the air from a standing start and land on two feet as stable as possible.

- Heiden Hop Test: Jump as far as possible with the uninjured leg and land on the injured leg. Your ability to stick the landing is indicative of good knee function.

- Isokinetic Testing: This is used to evaluate muscle strength. For the patellar tendon autograft, the injured leg should have at least 90% quadriceps strength of the uninjured leg, and equal hamstring strength.

My own rehab followed this general five-phase plan, however, the five-phase plan is very "vanilla," and the details do not give a real sense of what day-to-day rehab is like. I kept careful notes of what I did and how I felt throughout my rehab. What follows is a summary of those notes.

As someone who had never had surgery before, and rarely gets sick or suffers from long-term ailments, I was absolutely shocked at how beat up my knee was after surgery. I've had plenty of minor scrapes and setbacks including broken bones, muscle pulls, back spasms, and even Lyme disease, but none of these made me feel as helpless, made me suffer as much pain, and required as long of a rehab effort as ACL replacement surgery. Any previous accident or injury I incurred felt 100% within 6 to 12 weeks of normal rest and recovery. In contrast, the recovery from surgery required a consistent year-long effort, and I am not sure if/when the injured knee will ever feel completely normal. Even five years after surgery, I retain a small numb spot on the repaired knee, so that I rarely mistake it for the uninjured knee.

The improvement curve for rehab is like the classic learning curve – a great deal is achieved very early on, but every subsequent step of improvement takes longer and longer. I kept a fairly detailed journal of my rehab at the start, but naturally, as time went on and improvement slowed down, I made entries less often. There are a lot of notes in the first few days, then the notes taper off to weekly, and finally monthly. Here is a quantitative overview of how I felt during the yearlong rehab, where post-surgery is 0% and back-to-normal is 100%.

The first month, week by week:

| Week 1 – 10% | Week 2 – 20% | Week 3 – 30% | Week 4 – 40% |

And, the first year, month by month:

Month 1 – 40%	Month 2 – 60%	Month 3 – 75%	Month 4 – 80%
Month 5 – 84%	Month 6 – 87%	Month 7 – 90%	Month 8 – 92%
Month 9 – 94%	Month 10 – 95%	Month 11 – 96%	Month 12 – 97%

The rest of this chapter picks up the details of my story from the time I returned home from surgery through my rehabilitation. My rehab was smooth and successful, and typical for people who follow the program. You can use this diary to get a general sense of the physical and emotional challenges that you will face in your own rehab. Each patient's experience is different, but you will very likely share many of the experiences you read here.

Day 1

My surgery was early Friday morning March 9, 2012, and I was home by 2:30 PM. I agreed to a femoral nerve block before surgery because this allowed the anesthesiologist to minimize his use of drugs, and indeed, according to my surgeon, I breathed on my own throughout the procedure. After surgery, I woke up quickly and easily - at least that is what I remember. My wife tells me that once I started to wake up they allowed her to come see me, and while she and the doctor talked to me, she reports that I was slurring my speech and losing track of the conversation. As I struggled, she says that I kept shaking my head like a dog shakes off water after swimming, presumably in a vain effort to shake out the grogginess. She says it was very funny – like Wyle E Coyote shaking himself back to normal after being hit with a boulder. The nerve block effectively blocked all feeling in the front and sides of my leg. The back of my leg had sensation, but only the ankle and below had control and movement. Pain was minimal.

My leg was effectively dead, unable to bear any weight at all. It was as though I had a big plank stuck to my hip, with a very swollen hot center. When I woke up they offered me crutches, and I quickly hopped off to the bathroom. I was familiar with crutches from a broken fibula years earlier, so I moved quickly and easily. The nurses laughed with surprise when they saw me move with agility, and I was glad to be awake and alert.

Here is a picture of a leg two days after ACL replacement surgery. This is not a picture of my leg, but it looks very much like my leg did. I was so annoyed and distracted right after surgery, that I did not have the presence of mind to take any photos. A year later, I remembered to ask a friend to snap a few photos of his own leg after surgery. He obliged me; thanks Ben! Ben and I shared the same surgeon. Ben also had a patellar tendon autograft. Notice the vertical taped incision on the left inside of the right knee. Also, notice the small taped hole above the knee, on the lower right of the thigh. This is the hole through which a line is threaded that aligns and pulls the graft into place. Finally, note the difference in size between the healthy knee and the knee that was operated on. Ben is a good deal younger than I am, and the difference in his knees was less pronounced than mine.

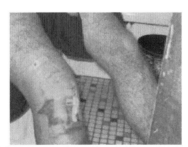

Swollen right leg, two days after ACL replacement surgery

The numbness was very frustrating. I longed desperately to get some feedback and know just how much pain I was in, but I would have to wait two more days. Meanwhile, at home, I lay down in the den with the CPM (continuous passive motion) machine that had been delivered earlier in the week.

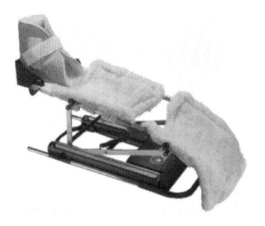

A Typical CPM Machine

A CPM machine bends your leg slowly and continuously up and down, something I could not do at all by myself. The goal of using the CPM is to get the knee bending up to 90 degrees within a few days, and more importantly to get the leg to straighten out to zero degrees or even lock out at -5 degrees. Getting the leg to straighten out as soon as possible is crucial to a positive long-term outcome. Leaving slack in the straightening for the first few weeks can result in a permanent loss of range of motion and inability or difficulty to later lock the leg.

It is not clear whether a CPM is necessary. Studies have not demonstrated whether long-term outcomes are better with or without a CPM. However, a CPM is the only way to do anything at all helpful in the first few days after surgery, and emotionally it feels great to be doing something. Some surgeons recommend that patients use the CPM just a few hours a day, others recommend up to 16 hours a day, and some say you can't use it enough in the early days - recommending even sleeping in it. I used the CPM as much as 18 hours a day at the start and continued using it less each day for two weeks. After ACL surgery, a CPM is typically used from one to three weeks.

With determination, I set the machine to 90 and -5 immediately. I was able to tolerate this accelerated pace because the nerve block prevented me from feeling any pain. Normally, you set the numbers lower (40 degrees) and work up to the limits of 90 and -5. My decision to jump to the maximum immediately was due to impatience - I needed to get back to work in a week and I was eager to get ahead of schedule.

The machine moved my dead leg up and down -- easily going to 90 degrees and -5 right away. Nonetheless, it was hard to sleep, and I would drag the leg in and out of the CPM every few hours just to change positions. Still, I loved that machine because it was the only way I could move the leg at all. After two more weeks, I developed a more sophisticated love/hate relationship with the CPM.

I also had a Cryo-Cuff, which is a pressurized ice pack that sits around the knee all the time. There is a valve connected to the pack from where the ice can be drained and refilled without having to remove the pack. The pack needs to be drained and refilled every 2-3 hours, or whenever you feel you need it colder. An insulated gallon container that stands nearby serves as the reservoir for the pack, and lasts for about 24 hours before having to be emptied and refilled. The Cryo-Cuff is a very convenient contraption.

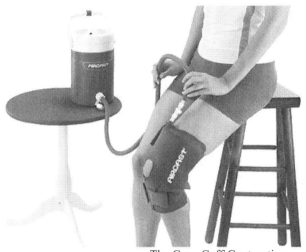

The Cryo-Cuff Contraption

Every two to three hours I would refresh the ice in the reservoir. This continuous pressure and ice treatment continued for many weeks, long after I finished with the CPM.

Day 2

I still hadn't taken any of the pain medication I had been given, because the nerve block was warding off any serious pain. Indeed, my whole leg was still mostly numb. I was so frustrated from not having any real feedback that I vowed not to take any pain medication, until I could feel just how bad off my knee was. The nerve block was supposed to wear off in anywhere from 18-36 hours, but mine had worn off only partially, and did not wear off completely until the third day.

I finally started to feel real pain later in the day especially in the patella itself when straightening the leg. With the renewed feeling in my leg, I began to regain some minimal control over bending the leg myself. I gritted my teeth at the pain but I was pleased to have any kind of feedback. It was Saturday - the day after surgery, and I felt things were improving. Normally on Saturday, I walk to services at our local synagogue, but I did not leave my bed or chair all day. Happily, a number of friends came to visit with me and I was very glad to see them. I sat with them in the living room, and the pain started to come in hard after they left.

At this point, I was also allowed to remove the dressing from the wound. Until now the knee was covered with a mummy wrap of gauze, underneath which were strips of tape over the incisions and holes. I figured that after unwinding all the gauze my leg would seem thinner, but I was mistaken. I had a watermelon for a knee. The normal shape and contours were completely indiscernible.

I used the CPM half the night. It was easier to sleep than the first night because of my regained muscle control from the disappearing nerve block. Overall, however, the second day was much worse than the first. The increasing pain, along with my more capable attempts to move the knee without the CPM, was a recipe for frustration. It was depressing to feel all that pain and to have such little control over the leg. I had no confidence at all that I would get back to work in a week. Why did I do this? Intellectually, I knew that cutting my leg open would temporarily set me back, however, I had no inkling how badly surgery would mangle my leg, and how quickly I would emotionally crumble from the helplessness and discomfort. I was not used to feeling helpless, and I did not like it.

Getting to the bathroom was a big challenge. Besides having to move on crutches, it was hard to bend the leg enough, without the help of the CPM, to be able to sit down. Still, I did not take any pain medication because the pain was physically, if not emotionally, bearable. I used the Cryo-Cuff all the time, including when I slept, but by the morning it was warm and not so effective.

At this point, I was still not able to lift my leg while lying flat on my back. It had been two days since the communication channels from my brain to my right leg seemed to be down, and I continuously tried and retried to send the leg a message to move. At some point, I changed positions to lie on my side, and I was happily surprised when my leg rose on cue. With my knee facing the wall, the leg moved upward toward the ceiling, something it would not do at all with my knee facing the ceiling. I was thrilled. It felt like the first time my dad let go of me riding a two-wheel bike and I kept going. It was that kind of positive thinking that got me out of my funk.

Day 3

The nerve block finally wore off completely, and I got real feedback. The knee was very stiff, but the CPM helped a lot by moving it for me continuously and loosening it up. I could get to the bathroom more easily, and I became able to lift my leg while lying on my back. This was absolutely impossible on day 2, and indeed I was quite surprised to see my leg move. I still had numbness completely around the knee, but the leg itself had regained feeling. The numbness around the knee is not due to the nerve block, but to collateral damage of local nerves during surgery. It took at least a year for most of this numbness to disappear, and it diminished slowly with the center of the numbness around the lower outside section of the knee. After four months the numb area was still the size of a playing card. After nine months, it was the size of a quarter, with minor numbness radiating outward. Five years later, a small numb stop remains, and will probably be permanent.

To protect the knee, you are supposed to wear a full leg brace, from upper thigh to your ankle, that theoretically protects the graft in the case of a fall. Indeed, some surgeons insist on wearing this brace to sleep, and when moving around anytime during the first six weeks. Some studies show that although the brace gives extra support and stability and helps avoid silly accidents and falls, it is not effective at protecting the graft in the event of a bad accident. Mostly, the brace is a reminder and an insurance policy, but it is not a magic shield.

I did not use the brace in bed for the first two days because my knee had been in the CPM, but on the third day I stopped using the CPM at night, so I finally wore the brace in bed. I hated the brace but I slept a lot better than the first two nights. The downside of giving up the nightly use of the CPM is that the leg is quite stiff by the morning.

I still had not left the house, spending most of my time lying down. Today I was able to move around more and believed for the first time that I would be able to return to work within a week. I still used the Cryo-Cuff all the time, and the swelling around my knee had diminished considerably. The knee looked more like a grapefruit than a melon.

I still had not used any painkillers, and the pain was so diminished compared to the second day, that I was sure I would never be using any. Was this the right decision? I am not sure, but I am glad I did it in retrospect. If I had loaded up on Vicodin during the first two days after surgery I would not have known how bad off I was, and I might have pushed too hard. In fact, I believe that part of the excessive pain the second day was because I had pushed too hard and too fast with the CPM on the first day due to the numbness of the nerve block.

The only real downside to avoiding the painkillers was the effect it had on my wife. I could not have survived the first few days without the loving care of my wife who left me books and lunch within reach, and called regularly to provide emotional support. She was the one who suffered the most from my stubbornness about the painkillers. During the second day and to a lesser extent the third day, I was depressed and I am sure I made her annoyed and uncomfortable with my moaning and complaining.

132

Perhaps it is a little selfish to avoid painkillers completely, but if I had used painkillers, I would never have developed an aversion to surgery, which I think is a very healthy emotional response. I believe that pain is a natural bodily response that builds healthy emotional responses. Artificially "managing" pain interferes with building these emotional responses. Not even nine long months of rehab are a substitute for these early pain memories. If you can stand the pain, I recommend confronting it because the long-term emotional benefits outweigh the short-term discomfort. I believe that the negative experience from the early pain may protect me from future injuries out of unconscious fear.

Day 4

Different doctors have different opinions, but mine allowed me to get rid of the crutches as soon as I could bear weight on the leg, although the brace would have to stay on for six weeks for protection. Some recommend crutches for longer, and are not as vigilant about the brace. It all has to do with protecting the graft and avoiding a second surgery at all costs – different approaches for the same purpose.

I was able to walk slightly without crutches and I marveled at how far I had come in just a few days. I no longer regretted the surgery. My ability and strength in performing leg lifts increased. I finally left the house for the first time and took a very slow walk down the block relying heavily on crutches. I was able to take a few steps without the crutches and I felt like I had come along way. I slept well without the brace, against doctor's orders. The Cryo-Cuff still got warm by morning, even when I refreshed it in the middle of the night.

Day 5

I could walk completely without crutches but I wore the brace. The knee got progressively looser, although it stiffened after sitting for a while with it bent.

My wife drove me to work. I was officially not allowed to drive because the damaged leg is my driving leg. I felt like I could almost drive myself, however, in an emergency the leg would not move quickly enough. I am allowed to drive when I can move the leg fast enough to avoid an emergency.

I had no scheduled lectures on my first day back to work, so I worked for a while in my office. I was able to climb stairs without crutches. I still used the CPM at least 10 hours a day at home, and I maintained the Cryo-Cuff both at home and at work. I slept peacefully again without the brace, but woke up at 1:00 AM with pain and impatience. I took some Advil, leaving the Vicodin unopened, and quickly got back to sleep.

Day 6

Improvement started to kick in strongly. I had more mobility, less pain, and less swelling. It was, however, always two steps forward and one step backward – the nature of any rehabilitation program. As I worked the leg harder, I developed new pains and aches. A burning started in my shin near the patella graft harvest.

Days 7 and 8

On day 2, I missed Saturday services but a week later, I walked to synagogue. I brought crutches but ended up carrying them. I walked very slowly but not too slowly to annoy my kind friends who picked me up to accompany me. The burning shin pain persisted but was less severe. Stiffness after sitting for a while continued for weeks, but overall, pain was much diminished.

Day 9

I felt much better at this point. I slept normally, without the brace, and with much less pain and much more mobility. I went to gym for the first time, lifted some weights for my arms, and rode 3.5 miles on a stationary bike to loosen up the knee. Getting back to work would not be any trouble after all.

Day 10

I returned to work without crutches. In a few days, I would be lecturing again and spending hours on my feet. I felt that I would be able to manage.

At this point, the daily changes in my condition were less perceptible, so I started keeping track of my progress weekly, rather than daily. And, after 16 weeks of rehab, I changed to monthly notes for the same reason. Although I had improved so much from how I felt after surgery, I still had many months to go before reaching 100%. It is remarkable both how fast I improved from a dead lump to a functioning human being, but how slowly I returned to full function.

As time went on, my strength increased, my balance and flexibility improved, my pain diminished, and my endurance and range of motion returned to normal. The great percentage of this improvement occurred early on, but a complete 100% recovery would take much longer. I kept reminding myself that Wes Welker had 80+ receptions in his first season back, nine months after surgery, but did not return to superstar stats of 120+ receptions until his second season back.

Week 2

I was walking without crutches, still using the CPM most days, and my quads were starting to fire. I could walk upstairs fine, but downstairs was harder. It was generally easier to push up on the bad knee than to support my weight on it while going down. Thus, as I would walk downstairs, my good leg would smash into each stair as my bad leg quit holding up my weight. If I tried to place the good leg down more softly, my bad leg would shake with weakness under the load it was bearing. This "leg shake" eventually disappeared completely but not until months more of rehab. One of the last things to get back to normal is a painless and smooth ability to support one's body weight on the injured knee while moving downwards. This is especially true with a patellar tendon replacement. Eventually, I developed a little plantar fasciitis, because of this repeated banging of my good heel into the stairs. This was one of many minor auxiliary injuries I would suffer while rehabbing the knee. Others included calf muscle pulls, tendinitis, and joint stiffness.

The range of motion in my knee was -5 to 100 degrees. The -5 was as good as necessary; I could effectively lock out my knee straight. Interestingly, later on, the -5 went back to +5 as my knee stiffened under the stresses of hard rehab, and later still, I returned to -5 as my patellar tendon became stronger and suppler. The 100 degrees would eventually increase to 180 but not until four months later, when I could finally pull my leg back and have the heel once again touch my butt.

Although my wife had arranged rides for me back and forth to work for the first six weeks, I felt ready to drive after a week, and she gave in after my two-week doctor visit. The doctor, sensible and conservative, did not recommend I drive myself until I was 100% sure I could react in an emergency and not hurt myself while doing so. If a child were to jump in front of my car, I needed to have the confidence to stop on a dime. Fortunately, I never had to test my reaction time. All my good friends who signed up to drive me back and forth to work got their good deed credit without having to leave home.

First Post Surgery Doctor Visit (2 weeks)

I saw the doctor two weeks after surgery so he could evaluate my progress. It was fortunate I hadn't seen him on day 2 when I was grouchy; I was in a much better mood after two weeks. I sat on the examination table with both legs dangling off the end. He said I looked great. I showed up carrying the brace rather than wearing it and he reminded me that I should wear it for 6 weeks – I hated the brace. He then removed the magic long blue suture than ran through my graft harvest. He wrapped the end of the suture that poked out of my knee around a scissor to get a good grip, and pulled firmly. Ideally, the suture just pulls out, but mine promptly broke. He wound up the remainder of the suture and tried again, eventually pulling out the whole thing. It felt good to have the suture out and the tape off – I wanted to get back to normal as soon as possible. He said I should start PT immediately, so I set up a schedule, with the first meeting immediately following my visit with the doctor. I would see Dr. Berkson again after six weeks.

Week 3

I began physical therapy twice a week. The goals were to reduce swelling and stiffness, increase range of motion from what was now about 120 degrees, improve balance, and regain strength. I was also encouraged to rub the scar, and slide the patella itself up and down and left to right. The skin does not feel normal after surgery. It is stiff and filled with scar tissue. It does not slide like normal skin. After a strong massage, you can feel the skin burn slightly, as the scar tissue "melts." It took months, but after a while the skin did feel normal once again.

The scars from the arthroscopic part of the surgery were now teeny holes and almost invisible. The scar from the patellar tendon graft was a thin three-inch line on the inside of the patella, which at this point was still raised thick and swollen, but after two more months was barely noticeable.

I still had burning shin pain and plenty of swelling. I had lost some muscle mass but much less than I could have lost. Ice and the Cryo-Cuff were recommended to manage swelling.

Week 4

I continued with physical therapy religiously doing my exercise sets at home or at the gym. I was less stiff, less swollen, but still needed regular ice applications. My range of motion was up to 150 degrees. Step downs were getting easier but still choppy. I did lots of stretching, strengthening, and balance drills. For example, I catch a ball over and over again while standing with one foot on a slightly unstable rubber balance mat. Balance workouts are the most difficult for me. This is mainly because I was never any good at these exercises before my injury. Even here, however, with practice comes improvement. By the end of my rehab, I had better balance than I ever had even pre-injury, and that improvement seems to have stuck. It may seem trivial, but I no longer stumble while putting on my shorts standing on one leg at a time.

Week 5

Until this week, there remained a noticeable limp in my gait, but now it was almost gone. Swelling had reduced almost completely and ice was needed only intermittently. According to my PT, the leg "looks good"; it had some normal shape again. My range of motion was up to 160 degrees (only slightly less than the good leg), and step-downs were almost normal. In general, the leg did not stiffen up as much after long periods of standing or rest.

At this point, my PT reduced our meetings down to weekly because I was successfully able to do the rehab at the gym and by myself. For insurance purposes, it is always good practice to save PT visits for when they are necessary. If you are conscientious and have learned and practiced your exercises, you do not need a PT to babysit you while you do your sets. Save the PT visits for when your PT needs to evaluate your progress, and/or teach you how to do new exercises, when that time comes.

Strengthening exercises vary from weight lifting to rubber band exercises to chair scoots. With the rubber band, one wraps a band around the ankle or mid-leg and you work against the force of the band to strengthen quads and hips. The chair scoots are the kind of thing a kid does for fun. One sits on a rolling chair and using only your legs, you pull yourself around a long hallway for two or three laps. The hallway is partly carpeted and partly tiled. It is always fun to get off the rug and have a few meters of easy tile floor sliding.

Week 6

I commuted to work by bike for the first time since surgery. This was against my doctor's recommendation. He was concerned that an accident or even an unexpected twist of the quick-release pedals could harm the still very fragile graft. This made a great deal of sense, but I am more comfortable on a bike than I am walking, so I felt no need to play it safe. If I was already walking without a brace, then I could bike too. I found that there was very little difference in commuting time, flexibility, or strength compared to my pre-surgery commute. I felt some very mild swelling afterwards, which I handled with ice. Biking, of course, puts very little stress on an ACL, so the fact that I could commute effectively with very few side effects after only six weeks is not surprising. Despite my success with bicycle commute, as my wife told me countless times, you should generally follow your doctor's recommendations.

I was using the brace intermittently at this point. I had almost no stiffness in the knee after standing for an hour lecturing in front of class, but prolonged time caused stiffness and swelling.

Second Post Surgery Doctor Visit (6 weeks)

Dr. Berkson examined my knee, performed the Lachman test, and proclaimed that the new ACL looked like it was doing its job. Furthermore, he said that my leg was strong and I was in the top 90% of patients in recovery, remarking that I looked more like an allograft recovery at this stage than a patellar tendon replacement. I was very happy about all this.

Six weeks was officially complete, and finally, the brace can go. Hurray! I never liked hobbling around in the brace and it rarely made me feel more sure-footed or stable. Most of the time, the brace accentuated my limp, and made me uncomfortable. It tended to slide down my pants, effectively hobbling my attempts to walk smoothly. Perhaps I was too lazy to strap the brace up correctly, but even when I was careful to do so, I found it a burden.

The idea of the brace is to keep the knee safe while the graft rebuilds. This rebuilding is called ligamentization. Indeed, the replacement graft weakens for the first six weeks and the tissue effectively dies before regaining blood supply. After six weeks the graft starts life once again as a ligament and begins to come alive. Why remove the brace when the graft is possibly at its very weakest? It has more to do with the chances for an accident than the weakness of the graft. After six weeks, most patients have regained much of their strength and balance, so the chances of falling are greatly reduced.

I ended up using the brace only about half the time, and mostly when I thought I needed a reminder to be careful. One of the advantages of the brace is that it allows a normal gait, whereas without it, the patient would surely develop a well pronounced limp that would subsequently have to be corrected. My brace, however, due to my sloppy adjusting, sometimes slipped down my leg, forcing my gait to be even more labored than it would have been without the brace. Adjusting and readjusting the brace carefully, especially after muscle growth, is a good plan, and one I should have followed more meticulously.

The post-operative brace is not intended to be worn while doing sports. It is primarily for protection and support. There is another "sports" brace that one can use after rehab is over for safety. It is also recommended for patients who do not opt for surgery. Indeed, I had one of these fitted before I elected to do surgery. This sports brace physically prevents you from twisting too much side to side. It is much more comfortable than the post-surgery brace and it is easier to get used to, but it too has issues. Using this brace makes you *feel* more limited than you actually are. Although it may physically prevent you from twisting severely, psychologically the effect is more pronounced. Some athletes feel that its use is too constraining. Others find the sense of safety comforting. In any case, be aware that this sports brace will *not* prevent an ACL injury. Mostly, it is a good reminder to be careful.

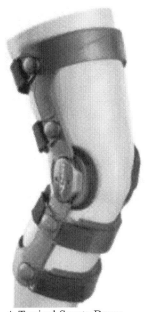 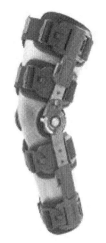

A Typical Sports Brace   The More Substantial Post-Op Brace

Week 7

I threw a Frisbee for the first time since surgery but avoided hip twisting, throwing mostly with my arm and shoulders. Really hard uncoiling twists that are required for long throws need to be avoided for months. Indeed, I was not sure I could make my body twist hard even if I tried. At this point, I had developed a self-protection memory that will take months to unlearn. Long after I was physically able to perform certain activities and motions, my body resisted my brain's messages. I noticed this especially for all actions that made my knee give out before surgery. Meanwhile, I kept going to the gym and meticulously repeating series after series of PT exercises.

After standing in class for a couple of hours, the knee still stiffened up, and got warm and painful. No more post-surgery brace, but the doctor recommends using the sports brace when I engage in activities I am not so confident about. I planned on wearing the sports brace at the end of semester Ultimate game, which would take place 8 weeks after surgery.

I was still not running at all yet, and although I was cycling, Dr. Berkson did not encourage that activity unless done on a stationary bike. I also started leg weight training in PT, doing leg presses of 70 pounds with each leg. It is important to maintain symmetry in rehab, and not just to exercise the injured side. After nine months, I was up to 120 pounds with each leg.

Week 8

I spent the week busy cycling, lifting, and doing various step exercises. The knee felt relaxed and almost normal after cycling. It still stiffened and swelled slightly after resting or standing. Despite the vast changes and improvements, my knee was still not normal.

I effectively walked/limped through the semester Ultimate game – the same game in which my unstable knee caused the re-injury that made me decide on surgery 4-5 months earlier. Running was completely out of the question, but I was able to throw fairly well even without a big twist. I wore the sports brace, walking back and forth across the field, and I handled my lack of mobility by playing offense for both sides.

The numbness in the knee was improving and I could feel much more. The actual numb spot was down at least 50% from about 15 squares inches to 6, centered below the patella and slightly toward the outside of the leg. The knee was less puffy and I could feel its natural contour that has been hiding behind tissue and fluid for two months. Climbing downstairs also continued to improve. Leg press was up to 90 pounds with the right leg, and 100 with the left.

Week 9

I tried to jog very slowly but I was not able to do it normally. I had a limp in my run and could not land hard and evenly. Running would have to wait for a few more weeks. Climbing downstairs, on the other hand, was almost normal, and step-down exercises were stronger with more smoothness and just a little "leg shake." After hard cycling or a light jog, there was still slight swelling and/or pain, but it disappeared soon after a couple of days. Leg presses and cycling continued. I was heading to Park City, Utah on a work-related trip for six weeks starting in week 10. My doctor recommended PT there 1-2 times per week.

Six weeks in Park City, Utah

Week 10

In Park City, land of the fit and fitter, I scheduled PT twice a week. I did my first real hike post-surgery. It was a 10-mile roundtrip, 1500 ft. elevation gain, from Mormon Flat near Park City to the border of Salt Lake City, along the route taken by the original Mormon settlers. I slipped once, hyperextending the bad knee and straining my patellar tendon, but fortunately the leg held up under the strain and the injury was minor. The weakness of my recovering leg caused repeated hard landings on the good leg throughout the hike. This exacerbated the plantar fasciitis in the good heel, and caused stiffness and swelling in the bad knee, but nothing that did not heal quickly.

Week 11

I worked with a variety of physical therapists in Park City, including a strength trainer who specializes in training college football players looking to make it to the NFL. Sessions with him were different from anything I had done before. He is used to extremely motivated and strong athletes. Usually, I feel I can push harder than my therapists want me to, but not with him.

One time, he held my legs in place while I kneeled down holding my upper body upright with my quads. I was supposed to lean forward maintaining control over my upper body. It was very difficult, partly because my right knee was so numb that it was awkward to kneel, and partly because it was challenging just to hold the position. I was ready to quit when he said, "Okay nice job, now hold it for just 30 more seconds." The next 30 seconds were excruciating and took all of my will power not to give up.

This trainer taught me lots of exercises I had never tried before, as well as plenty of standard strengthening exercises, including: hip abduction and adduction, high step-ups and step-downs with weights, one legged balance with/without eye turns and balance ball, lunges, single leg presses, single calf presses, hamstring curls, "clamshells" with rubber band pulling my knees together, leg slides with weights, and various other balancing exercises. Hamstring strengthening was the only thing that made me sore, but interestingly, after the hamstring exercises, my step-downs were without any leg shake whatsoever for the first time after surgery.

Balance and proprioception are a big challenge for me. Even before my injury I used to stumble when putting on shorts while standing on one foot. We did some serious work on this, including an exercise where I had to stand on one foot on an unstable balance pad, while he pulled my knee to the side with a bungee cord. Sometimes, I felt he was born to work in a medieval dungeon.

After a long day of lecturing for four straight hours, my knee still stiffened but it got loose fast. Serious stiffening was not a regular normal end of day event like it used to be. I felt that I would be ready to run in one or two weeks.

145

My range of motion in extension was 3-4 degrees less than the good leg. We worked on that and it improved slowly, but I had mild pain in the patellar tendon when attempting to completely extend my right leg. This inability to fully extend the leg without pain was not apparent in the first two months of recovery, and I did not regain full painless extension until after 10 months.

My gait, three months after surgery, was completely normal with no limp or hitch. I took a solo hiking trip to Arches National Park for the weekend where I hiked Fisher Towers and Delicate Arch. Fisher Towers is located a few miles outside of Arches National Park and a 7-mile long walk from the nice resort I stayed at on the Colorado River. The "towers" are beautiful red sandstone 1000-foot spires, popular with climbers. The hike winds around the towers for 4-5 miles with mild elevation gain.

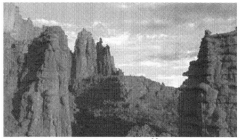

Fisher Towers[32]

There are some steep drop-offs and a ladder in one place to help navigate the through the cliffs, but overall it is a mild pleasant hike. The trail is easy to follow, but somehow, I got lost right at the start, adding a couple of miles to my trip as I wandered in and out of various gulches masquerading as trails. I finally got back on the trail after I realized that walking *away* from the cliffs behind me was not likely to be correct – duh!

---

[32] Public domain image from Wikipedia

I guess I was nervous about hiking solo in the middle of nowhere with a mediocre knee, because I got lost again right after descending the ladder. Here, somehow I scrambled forward for a half a mile and found myself on a very steep ledge with nowhere to go except backwards. I cleverly deduced that the last half mile had not been the trail. I backtracked to find the point where I had lost the trail at the bottom of the ladder. Normally, I never would have missed the trail; in hindsight, I seemed distracted.

Back on the trail, I caught up to a local who was admiring the views. She had grown up in a small village nearby called Castle Valley, and had hiked this trail dozens of times. I asked her about her home because this area is wilderness and there is very little civilization. She confirmed that her village was nothing more than a few roads, a bunch of homes, a tiny post office and town office, a small bed and breakfast, and a general store – no traffic lights, no hardware store, and virtually no retail or local business. She described her home as a beautiful remote desert spot surrounded by mountains and the Colorado River.

She led the way back to the trailhead, which took almost two hours less than the way in for me. It was easy to avoid getting lost by simply following her back. The next day I drove the 15 miles to Arches National Park and hiked all day including a trip to the famous Delicate Arch. The hike to Delicate Arch is routine; thousands of people do it every year. It starts on a wide dirt trail and eventually crosses some long slabs of rock where cairns mark the trail. The total length of the hike is no more than two miles with a few hundred feet of elevation gain.

Amazingly, I got lost here too, but this time my distraction was serendipitous. Although there were hundreds of people hiking near me, the slick-rock slabs are gigantic, and people spread out. Moreover, there are dozens of little side trails with their own cairns. Nonetheless, before I knew it, the cairns started to disappear along with the people. Eventually I lost sight of every other hiker. It is perhaps understandable to get lost at Fisher Towers, a much less popular site, where I saw only one other hiker the whole morning, but getting lost at Delicate Arch really feels impossible.

As I was about to give up and backtrack, I got my first glimpse of the arch itself – and headed directly toward it. I was making my own trail, but the occasional appearance of an isolated cairn let me know that others had surely come this way before.

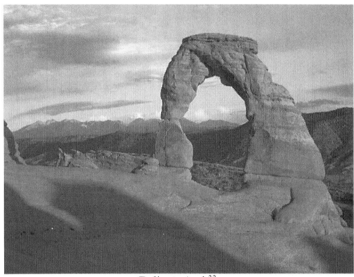

Delicate Arch[33]

Except for no people around me, everything was going smoothly as I aimed toward the arch. Suddenly, however, there was nowhere to go. The straight line to the arch would need to cross over a 1000-foot drop that spanned about a quarter mile. Now I understood why nobody else was here. The actual trail winds around the north of the arch avoiding this cliff. I hiked northward along the cliff finally finding an easy way down over some sand to the rock slabs

---

[33] Image in public domain from Wikipedia

below and a clear path eastward to the arch. Still there were no other people in sight, so I was slightly on alert.

The path to the arch runs along a hump of slick-rock about 100 meters wide and 400 meters long. The right side of the hump drops off 1000 feet straight down into the abyss I had seen from the other side a few minutes earlier. The left side of the hump drops into a bowl about 400 feet deep and the same distance across. The hump narrows to less than 10 meters as you approach the arch more closely. In the picture, the bowl is between the photographer and the arch, with the abyss behind the arch. I was approaching from the right side of the photograph in line with the arch.

At this point I finally saw all the other hikers to my left, above the bowl on the top of a bluff. Their view of the arch is exactly what you see in this picture – looking southward. A few of the hikers had scrambled down around the east side of the bowl and were approaching parallel to the arch heading west directly towards me. All of us got to stand underneath the arch, but I was shocked at how steep the drop off was. I had thought that this arch sits in the middle of a flat empty desert, having seen its image so many different times including every Utah license plate. In fact, the arch sits on a thin hump of rock between a 1000-foot cliff, and a 400-foot bowl. Usually, the National Park Service is overprotective of visitors, bombarding hikers with warnings and disclaimers for even the mildest danger. Not so here.

Elderly, children, and sneaker-clad novices all hike to Delicate Arch. I am surprised that there are no accidents considering the danger and the lack of experience of some of the hikers. Still, if you do stay on the trail and do not wander from the viewing area, there is no danger at all.

The viewing area, which I never reached, is just a couple hundred meters away from the arch, and provides a safe vantage point. I thought that perhaps there are all sorts of warnings at the viewing area about not hiking down toward the arch, and that I saw nothing because I was off-trail. But I confirmed the lack of any signs at the viewing area of the main trail when I did this hike with my wife the "right" way, five years later.

The arch is truly spectacular whether or not you scramble down to touch it. I was lucky to have gotten lost. If I had been at the normal viewing point, I would never have ventured down along the north side of the bowl and then westward to the arch. It requires sure-footing and excellent balance not to fall into the bowl, and my knee was not ready for that pressure. The scramble around the bowl is much scarier than the route I took to the arch. I saw one or two hikers, who had attempted the scramble, frozen in fear. Afraid that they would slip into the bowl, they were neither able to continue toward the arch, nor to turn back up to the viewing point. Eventually, some sure-footed fearless hikers ventured out to help them. I remained safely on the other side of the arch from the viewing point, preferring to tell my family personally about this hike, rather than have them hear in the news about their idiot loved one falling off a cliff.

Week 12

My leg extension continued to progress until I had just one or two degrees more until I could lock the knee with no pain. I threw a golf disc for the first time since surgery. Unlike Ultimate, a golf disc throw requires more hip rotation and knee flex. It was too early for me to let myself go, and my instinct to overprotect the knee caused my throw to be about 75 feet shorter than normal. I was now driving the disc only 200-260 feet, which was terribly frustrating. This loss of muscle memory would remain a problem months later.

150

I had good kneecap mobility – I could slide it up and down and left and right. The only swelling that remained was very mild in the lower inside half of the patella at the joint with the tendon. Swelling in the upper left, near the quadriceps, was gone. I could not yet run more than a few steps without pain and a slight limp. The knee was not strong enough to manage the shock of landing full force on one leg. Three months after ACL surgery is early for running, so that was normal.

Week 13

My extension continued to improve, as did my strength. The numb spot, isolated mostly to lower outside of knee, was about the size of a playing card. This numbness continued to lessen and shrink but was still noticeable a year after surgery. I had my last Park City physical therapy appointment and would not return to PT until after my four-month checkup.

My family came out to visit me my last week in Utah, and we did a lot of hiking, in lieu of physical therapy. The two older boys came out first, and we took a 12-mile roundtrip walk from my home in Park City to the Olympic ski-jump site. We later took a short hike on the famous Salt Flats, 150 miles west of Salt Lake. I finished my work at the University later that week, and my wife and my youngest son joined us for a trip to Zion National Park.

We did a number of hikes, two of which are worth reporting:

a. Angels Landing, a famous and popular hike in Zion National Park, and

b. Kanarra Creek Canyon, a local slot canyon outside Zion.

Angels Landing rises 1500 feet over the Zion canyon floor. The trail winds up switchbacks for two miles to Scout's Lookout, and then continues a half-mile eastward over a long thin finger of land with steep cliffs on the north and south sides. This thin ridge ranges in

151

width from four to 20 feet, with a 1000-foot drop on the north side and 600 feet on the south. People do fall off but it is rare; and whether you fall off the north or south side doesn't really matter. The National Park Service erected chains for hikers to hold onto in order to make the hike safer.

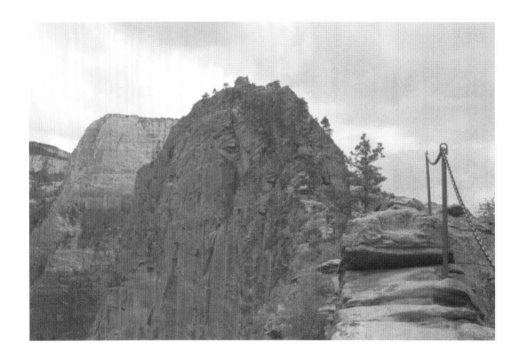

The Saddle of Angel's Landing, Zion National Park[34]

After so many weeks of rehab, my hiking strength felt normal, but my confidence level was not. I had done this hike 10 years earlier without a care and rarely touched the chains. It had taken me then about 2.5 hours without rushing. This time it took me about four hours and I held on to almost every section of chain meticulously watching every step I took. I had never

[34] Released by Daniel Smith into Public Domain

before felt fear or nervousness about heights and even though I was still pretty sure-footed, I could not completely put aside my fear of stumbling and falling into oblivion. This situation was particularly disturbing since I was the one in the group expected to help others who might get nervous. I was the one who was supposed to have confidence to spare and share.

The bottom line was that I did not feel as agile and spry as I had a decade earlier. My confidence was more broken than my balance and my knee. Once again, I was reminded that my rehab was going to have to be physical *and* emotional.

The Kanarra Creek slot canyon outside Zion is much less well known than its cousin's famous Narrows to the southeast. It is a family hike for sure: 2-3 miles through a beautiful slot canyon with only one or two difficult obstacles.

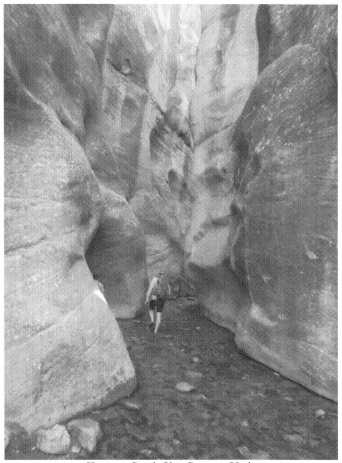

Kanarra Creek Slot Canyon, Utah

Our hiking group included five adults and four children ranging in age from 10 to 18. The photo below shows the first obstacle – a ten-foot waterfall around a wedged boulder. Notice the log propped up on the right that hikers use to scramble around the waterfall. If you look very carefully you will also see a short yellow climbing line I tied in place to allow the kids to hold on as they ascended. I climbed up and down the log a number of times helping the children feel comfortable and safe, but like Angel's Landing, I did not have the same confidence in myself as I did before my knee injury.

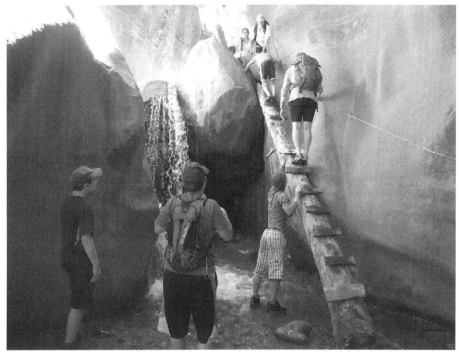

Climbing around a waterfall in Kanarra Creek Slot Canyon – me last on the ladder

This lack of confidence invaded everything physical that I tried to do. I found that I could not pull through my disc golf throw with any real conviction. My body seemed to instinctively prevent me from making the hard twist I needed for a successful throw. I wore my sports brace, thinking this might help me psychologically, if not also protect the knee physically. However, I still felt nervous that a hard pull would reinjure the new graft, and I was unable to throw as hard as I used to. Maybe all this mental hesitation was healthy. After all, it was less than four months after surgery, and the graft was still not ready to handle a full twisting effort.

155

Hard hiking was fine and encouraged, but not yet hard twisting. This self-protection, however, stayed with me a long time after my graft was physically able to handle the stress of full twisting. It was not until at least ten months after surgery that I was able to work through this mental/emotional aspect of the recovery more completely.

Four-Month Checkup – half way there

I returned from my trip to Utah 14 weeks after surgery, just in time for my four-month checkup with Dr. Berkson. The knee looked perfect and I was given the thumbs-up to start running, but still no twisting. My physical therapy visits were down to once in two weeks. My exercises were more dynamic including skipping, bounding, and hopping. The skin around the knee was less thick and rigid; it slid almost as well as the skin on the good knee. The patellar tendon scar was almost invisible. The patella itself moved easily and smoothly. The knee clicked occasionally but with no pain or adverse effects. My next, and hopefully last, appointment with Dr. Berkson, would be in three months, seven months after surgery.

Weeks 15-16

I continued physical therapy once every two weeks and started hopping exercises. I hopped from side to side and front to back over and over. I skipped, jogged, and jumped. I had much less "bounce" in the injured leg – even simple skipping felt abnormal. Jogging was better than hopping and skipping. With jogging there is a hard planting and push off, but not the same repeated fast springing that is necessary with hopping. The leg had plenty of strength, but it hurt when I tried to "spring" up and land. I continued to do lots of cycling, about 400-500 miles a month. I also hiked regularly, climbing up and down a half dozen 300-foot hills at the Blue Hills

Reservation in Canton over a distance of 3-4 miles, once a week. I was able to bowl and enjoy normal casual recreation without any noticeable side effects.

Month 5 – (weeks 17-20)

Physical therapy continued once every two weeks. I could jog up to a half mile, and the knee felt "thinner" and more flexible. There was almost no swelling or puffiness at all even after running, but there was slight stiffness. Hopping felt more normal. As far as flexibility goes, I could finally pull my leg back and touch my heel to my butt, but I needed to pull hard to do it. The numb spot was still significant, centered below the kneecap and slightly toward the outside of the knee. The numbness has no effect on anything expect that kneeling feels funny.

Month 6 – (weeks 21-24)

I was now running a mile at about a 9-minute pace – not bad. When I was in my 20s I used to run 7:30 miles for 4-5 miles. When I was 27, I ran a 47-minute 10k without any training, but even with a healthy knee, I couldn't keep up that pace today, so my goal was to get the pace down to 8:30 and I would be quite satisfied. The knee was still numb, but the degree of numbness is diminishing, and the size of the numb spot is shrinking.

I played a round of disc golf at my home course at Borderland State Park for the first time in over a year. My usual score had been 52, two under par; my goal was 60 and I shot a 56 despite drives that were generally shorter than before. I was very encouraged by this. My early attempts at disc golf a month ago were much worse. Then, I had been more nervous and hesitant about twisting and I was unable to play as well. It is still a long way from 56 to an average of

52. I continued to do all sorts of hip strengthening exercises – like sidestepping with bands around ankles. And of course, leg presses and stretching.

Month 7 – (weeks 25-28)

For general conditioning, I continued to run a mile, and I returned to my normal 20-mile roundtrip bicycle commute. I did the leg press and hamstring curls for strength, and a few hip rotation exercises for balance and stability. The hip exercises required standing on one leg, while I rotated my hips and move the other leg with and without resistance in various directions.

My PT visits were now only once every three weeks. The knee continued to "thin out" but I could not completely lock the leg straight without some pain. I got to about zero degrees easily without any pain, but there was mild pain and I felt like something was in the way when I pushed to -5 degrees. I started to aggressively massage the patellar tendon, which felt great. There was a healthy burning sensation as the scar tissue broke up.

Month 8 – (weeks 29-32)

I was finally able to run up to two miles every few days, in addition to the 20 miles a day of cycling. My patellar tendon was more pliable and thinner, but I still could not lock my leg to -5 degrees without some pain. Also, hopping hard caused minor pain. Overall, everything continued to improve with the occasional setback of new injuries from pushing too hard. The plantar fasciitis and sore Achilles tendon in my good (left) foot that I developed from pushing and compensating too hard were almost all gone. I occasionally pulled a calf muscle or sustained another minor injury, but these heeled quickly.

My last scheduled PT visit was immediately followed by a final meeting with Dr. Berkson, who evaluated my status. We did a one-foot bend from a stair dropping the other foot to the floor slowly. My good leg was noticeably better at doing this, and the bad leg bent inwards if/when I lost my balance. This simulated potential for re-injury. It is the collection of leg, hip, and abdominal muscles that ultimately stabilize the knee making it easy for the ACL to do its job. If the knee bends inwards with stress, then a severe force could push the ACL beyond the 450 pounds it can handle.

At this point, the graft itself was almost at full strength, so once I finished the rehab I was ready to go back to sports 100%. Dr. Berkson recommended one more PT visit with the goal of getting a regiment of exercises I would stick to for a few more months to supplement my running and cycling. I never scheduled that last PT visit.

Month 9 – (weeks 33-36)

I pretty much went back to my normal activities. I still had mild recurring pain in the knee especially after running and when trying to hyperextend (locking out). I continued to massage the patellar tendon on, around, and below kneecap to break up the scar tissue. With each massage, the knee felt more flexible and suppler, and even mild pain would diminish after massaging. I could run two miles at about an 8:40 pace, and my leg press was 120 pounds on each leg. I had no swelling, but there was still slight warmth after running. A little numbness remained over the kneecap and the right outside area of the knee, but overall sensation was generally returning. It still felt funny kneeling – but kneeling caused no pain and there was no pain when I massaged the knee.

Month 10 – (weeks 37-40)

There was much less pain when hyper-extending; I could almost lock out the knee normally. For the first time, I could believe that someday I might not be able to tell which leg was operated on. The numbness was diminished, and I could finally kneel and feel somewhat normal on the right knee. The heel to butt pull was easy and completely normal – as easy as the good leg. There was still some pain and warmth in the knee after running but it disappeared quickly.

I pulled a calf muscle rehabbing – something I also did in month 6. I could not walk well for a couple of days and could not run for two weeks, but after that I was fine again. Mentally, I was protecting my motion much less than I had automatically been doing for months. The knee felt about 98% healthy, however, I had returned to only about 80% of my pre-surgery form at sports. My disc golf throw was still 20% less far, and I did not jump as smoothly and easily as I used to in basketball or Ultimate.

Month 11 – (weeks 41 – 44)

I could hyperextend and lock almost normally with no pain, and the pain after running was minimal. I finally could pass the "test" of running for 15 minutes and then standing on my reconstructed leg without any wobble. I felt I was close to normal again.

It was exactly one year ago when my knee gave out in the end of semester Ultimate game. That accident tore my meniscus, and led to my decision to have surgery for the torn ACL. A year later, I played again. I could run, throw, pivot, and jump, but I was not yet 100%. Ironically, I strained my good knee while playing Ultimate, causing a slight twinge for a few days when climbing stairs. This minor injury was enough to make me momentarily forget which knee was the one with ACL replacement. At this time, there was no visual distinction between the good knee and the bad knee; even the scar was hardly visible. I could not feel any difference between the knees except for the slight numbness on the lower outside of the injured knee; the skin around the patellar tendon of the repaired knee was thin and soft.

Despite the fact that I felt almost normal again, it continued to be a long process to regain my pre-surgery form and agility. My ability to cut quickly and to jump naturally was not quite there yet. Also, mentally, I still did not yet completely trust the leg. These mental and physical challenges took another year, at which point there was no remaining effects of the surgery.

After a Year Plus

Long after the ACL got to 100% strength and there was no pain left due to the replacement, there was a lot more rehab needed, due to the trauma to the patellar tendon. I did not realize just how much time and effort it would take for me to regain the normal function and strength in my knee due to the secondary damage to my patellar tendon. In particular, holding my body weight bent on the bad leg, and stepping down with the good leg was an action I could not do smoothly for months. Even after nine months, hopping down stairs on the bad leg was mildly painful.

A year after surgery, I felt like full recovery was just a matter of time and patience. The numb spot on my knee continued to recede slowly to approximately the size of a quarter. The slight pain under the patella after jumping and sprinting disappears quickly. My performance at sports as far as strength and agility is concerned continued to converge (and even surpass) my pre-surgery levels.

Two years after surgery, the numb spot was down to a dime-sized area just below and outside the patella. Kneeling feels almost normal, the leg was able to straighten completely without any pain, and I could perform as well or better in any sport than I did before the injury. I dream one day to be able to say that I cannot quite remember which leg is the injured one.

Five years after surgery, the numb spot is still there, but the repaired knee feels like new. And, indeed, I did once briefly forget which knee had had the surgery. This happened when the good knee incurred a mild strain injury. Overall, I am very glad I underwent the procedure.

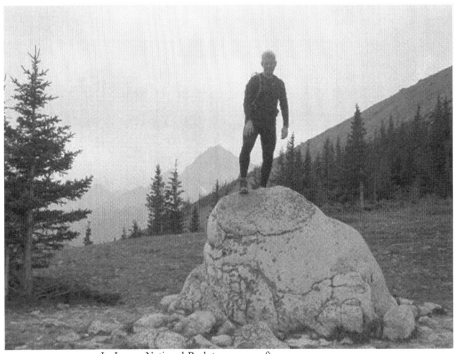

In Jasper National Park two years after surgery

Chapter 6 – Patient Interviews and Stories

"Example is not the main thing in influencing others. It is the only thing."

Albert Schweitzer, physician and philosopher

Each and every ACL story is different. It is important to familiarize yourself with as many people's experiences as you can. If all your information comes from merely one friend's story, you will likely construct many myths regarding ACL injuries. I heard and read lots of "common wisdom" that turned out to be wrong. I wished I had had a medley of stories to read through when I was trying to determine

a. whether or not I had torn my ACL, and

b. what to do about it when I found out that it was torn.

Wes Welker, Tiger Woods, and Derrick Rose all injured their ACLs without external contact. Tom Brady, on the other hand, tore his ACL when a defender rolled onto his planted front leg as he was about to throw. An acute external force is a common way for ACL tears to occur but not the most common. Indeed, the most common way for an athlete to tear his/her ACL is via a sudden deceleration of the leg often accompanied by sharp planting and twisting.

Just as the injuries that cause a torn ACL differ widely, so do the decision processes regarding treatment and the subsequent timeline for surgery. My own story is one of thousands. It was two months before my tear was diagnosed and confirmed, four months more before I decide to have surgery, and three more months before the surgery itself. Tiger Woods delayed his surgery and won the 2008 US Open with a torn ACL. Other athletes like Welker and Rose moved very quickly toward surgery waiting just enough time to let the symptoms of the original injury dissipate.

Besides the timeline and nature of the injury, athletes differ in age, sport, gender, and level of performance. The pain at the time of injury and the ease and success of the rehab also vary. Some people return to their sports better than they were before their injuries. Others suffer from recurrent pain, limited range of motion, and suboptimal performance. And although almost every ACL tear requires surgical repair for a complete return to competitive sports, in some rare cases, people manage fine without surgery, especially with a partially torn ACL.

This chapter presents a large variety of scenarios for a torn ACL and the subsequent treatment decision and rehab process. You will read how different people react to similar challenges. Hopefully, you can find someone like yourself in this chapter, and even if you cannot, there is a great deal to learn from these stories. I included a variety of ages, athletic skill, and gender. I tried to highlight different treatment decisions and outcomes. There are so many different things that make each person's story unique.

Some of the stories were told to me personally and others were posted on the Internet. Still others are a composite of a number of different people. I left narratives in first person with minimal editing to allow a person's style and personality to show. Other stories or composites are in third person, and generally shorter and less personal. You can find further patient cases on the Internet[35]as well as a number of "never-say-die" testaments from both amateur and professional athletes.[36]

To gather personal narratives, I sent people the letter below. I enjoyed reading different people's experiences as I hope you will, but more importantly, I learned a great deal from the examples they presented. When you are the patient, it is hard to imagine a different experience from the one you are having.

---

[35] http://ismoc.net/knee/patient1.html
[36] http://yeskneecan.com/2009/06/16/recent-famous-athletes-w-torn-acls/

Dear Friends,

I am currently working on a book about my experience with ACL surgery, with the support of my surgeon. I hope the book will be a useful guide for the 150,000 plus athletes each year who tear their ACLs.

I plan to dedicate one of the chapters in the book to people's stories, so the reader will be able to find someone like him/her self, and thereby be able to make a clear decision about what he/she wants to do with his/her own injury.

If you would like to tell me your story, I have listed some questions below to guide you, but feel free to focus on whatever aspects of your experience you prefer. You can answer the questions one by one, or just tell your story straight. I'll edit what you write but will not fiddle too much with your content or style. I will not use your name unless you give me explicit permission to do so, and I'll let you see what I plan to publish so you can approve it before publication.

Name: Gender: Age at Time for Injury:

1. Would you rather remain anonymous in the book?
2. How did you injure your knee? How old were you? What were you doing exactly? Try to tell the story briefly with as many details as you can remember.
3. How did you find out the ACL was torn? Did you get an MRI, an examination? How long did it take to diagnose the tear?
4. Did you decide on surgery?
5. How long between diagnosis and surgery?

6. Did you spend a long time deciding about surgery?

7. What kind of graft? How did you decide this?

8. Did you use pain medication? How bad was the pain after surgery?

9. Did you have a nerve block?

10. To the best of your recall, regarding your ability to move and need for crutches, drivers or other assistance, what was your experience in the first week? Two weeks? a month? Three months? One year?

11. Were you careful about your rehab and PT? How long did PT and rehab last?

12. Whether or not you choose surgery, did you ever have any episodes of instability, where your knee "gave out" after your injury?

13. Can you tell the difference now long term (how long?) between the two knees?

14. Did you have subsequent complications to the same knee or other knee? Please describe.

15. What advice would you give to someone regarding a torn ACL?

16. Anything else you would like to add?

Note that in each story, the age indicated is at time of injury. Any number of years may have passed from the time of injury to the time of the writing.

Jordan, 26-year-old Male

I was playing basketball in a church basement basketball court in Lewiston Maine in 1981, in my fourth year of medical school at Boston University. I was doing a one month rotation working in a hospital based clinic run by a small group of family practice residents in a program run by the Central Maine Medical Center.

One evening after work, I was invited to play basketball on a pick-up team. Toward the end of the evening, I found myself with a problem. The problem, which I literally ran into, was that this basement court had the basketball hoops mounted on the wall at each end with no room to stop or turn after doing a lay-up. I recall driving toward the hoop, launching the ball, and planting one foot in time to not smash into the wall. Needing to stop, turn, and pivot within an area of about six inches, I felt my left knee go crunch and I landed in a heap.

We were about a quarter mile from the hospital where I worked in the family practice clinic and from where I lived in an old Nursing dorm attached to the hospital. I proceeded to hobble over to the emergency room after my injury, where they briefly saw me, perhaps did a plain X-Ray, gave me ice and crutches, and sent me off to bed.

The next morning, I recall seeing a local young Lewiston orthopedic surgeon. After examining my tender, swollen left knee, he reported thinking that I had torn the meniscus cartilage and that he could remove the damaged tissue with his trusty arthroscope. He said that I would then be nearly as good as new. There were no MRIs and the CT images were poor at that time.

After speaking with my family in the Boston area and one of their orthopedists, I proceeded to have this surgery in Lewiston the next day or two. I do not recall the surgeon's name. After receiving a spinal anesthesia and the scope, he reported that the knee cartilage looked healthy, but that the ACL was a little frayed. After flushing blood clots, he finished up, and I hobbled across the hospital to my dorm room bed, returning home the next day on a bus.

I recall hobbling around on crutches for a week, then slowly beginning to walk, returning to work, and approximately a week later starting to run again. I soon resumed regular physical activities including a lot of bicycling, both local rides to different hospitals and some 50 to 100 mile recreational rides. I also played basketball, went downhill skiing, and enjoyed occasional games of squash.

Within two years of this basketball episode, I ran my first Boston Marathon in about 4 hours 10 minutes. I enjoyed it so much that I continued doing the slow run on a mostly annual basis, never getting an official number, but showing up for a fun day.

The twist comes about eight to ten years after my original injury. One year after running the Boston Marathon, my left knee had become a little swollen and painful. I took a week or two off from all exercise. One morning I remember hobbling around the halls of Goddard Hospital in Stoughton on my morning rounds with my Goddard Medical group. An orthopedist in the group, Bill Sullivan, saw my style of gait, took me into the ER, and after examining me, said he believed I had no ACL in my left knee. A few days later an MRI confirmed his suspicion. It seemed that I was an active pediatrician with no ACL in my left knee, apparently due to an injury almost 10 years earlier. I had never limited myself from doing any physical activities, nor did I ever have any joint complaints other than the several days in Maine immediately after the basketball injury in 1981. I had been functioning normally for ten years without an ACL in my left knee.

After my knee swelling resolved I discussed possible courses of action. With no history of knee complaints, I was told that not repairing my torn/missing left ACL was an option. I was told there was a study of US Marines comparing two groups with ACL tears, one with repair and the other without. After ten years, their soldiering abilities were the same! At approximately age 40 I decided not to undergo surgical repair.

I recall seeing an orthopedist, Dr. Bunch at the Baptist, for a second opinion about five years later. He was hesitant to recommend surgery, but instead had me fitted with a lightweight custom brace. He suggested I wear it for basketball, skiing, squash, etc. and that if I was unable to do any of these sports, then he would do the surgery. A year after, he moved to California! Oh well.

I am now 59 with two wonderful grown daughters. As I age, I continue to love sports and exercise. Now I have an asymmetric running gait, a leg length discrepancy, and have had recurrent unilateral lower back pain. Nonetheless, I stay active, including biking, sailing on the ocean, and still running the Boston Marathon annually, but with more difficulty each year.

I have done a regular morning Boot-Camp for the past five years at Elite Gym in Stoughton. Whenever I can participate in the groups led by Larry and Bernadette, I have hardly ever any low back pain/strain. I have recently been examined by one of the Gym PT owners, Keith, who sees my asymmetric gait. He wonders if having an ACL replacement surgery may decrease future damage to that knee as well as to the opposite knee.

I do not want to ever need a knee replacement. I want to continue to run the Boston Marathon, to ski, to hike the Appalachian Trail from Georgia to Maine, and maybe someday to play basketball again, all this at least until I am 85. After all, I did not beat icon Johnny Kelly in the Boston Marathon until he was in his 80's.

Should I have an ACL replacement now before it is too late? I do not know. Any opinions?

Kathy, 20-year-old Female

I had my first ACL repaired 27 years ago while I was in college. I tore it playing indoor soccer. There was a slight noise at the time of injury, and the knee felt "loose," but it did not swell terribly nor did it hurt very badly. I had a great sports surgeon repair it within a week of the injury. This was before arthroscopic surgery. They took a tendon from my thigh and attached it in place of the torn ACL. I have a big scar but it really held out.

I was in the hospital for a week and in a bent leg cast for three months. I went through physical therapy immediately afterwards starting with a very skinny leg. I worked hard and suffered with a limp for about four months, but the leg came back pretty quickly.

Twenty-three years later, I tore the other ACL, again playing soccer. After compensating for the injured knee for years, my "good" knee gave out when I planted the foot hard and scored a goal. This time it made a popping noise and swelled up immediately. I had physical therapy for two weeks before surgery, and had surgery in Waltham where they operate on lot of New England Patriots and other pro athletes. This time, the new ACL graft did not come from my thigh but from an Achilles tendon from a cadaver. I had outpatient day surgery and went home pumped with major pain killers and a brace. I immediately began using the CPM (continuous passive motion) machine and continued for two weeks, to obtain full range of motion.

Two days after surgery I began physical therapy again. It was very painful and arduous. It took about a year for my strength, range of motion, and especially my balance to feel normal again. Still, the surgery and rehab was much better than the experience of some of my friends who elected not to have surgery. A few of them had many problems.

Tifara, 17-year-old Female

My career-ending soccer injury occurred on October 7, 2010 when I was 17, and a senior at the Maimonides School in Brookline. It happened during a game in my final season of varsity soccer. Midway through the first half of the game, I stole the ball from the opposing team, and ran with it across the field. I could feel the adrenaline rush and all the pressure that was on me as I was gaining speed toward the goal. A few yards from the net, I could hear my teammates yelling, "Shoot, shoot!" As I was about to attempt to score, one of the opposing defenders (twice my size) came running toward me. She bumped against me so hard that I was knocked off my feet and in midair I felt something in my left knee pop or crunch (can't remember which cereal sound it made). When I hit the ground, I was in pain and I knew something was wrong. I was unable to get up and my coach and teammates crowded around me. It was soon clear that I was injured, so two of my teammates supported me as I hopped off the field on my right foot, avoiding any pressure on my injured leg.

As I sat helplessly on the sidelines watching the game continue, I felt pain both physically and mentally. The pain in my leg was intermittent but sharp, and I knew to my dismay that I would not be able to finish this game. After I had endured about a half hour of pain, my dad, who had come to see an exciting game, drove me to the ER, amid excitement he hadn't planned. The doctors determined that there were no broken bones, which at the time seemed hopeful. But I was not home free. I was in fact tentatively diagnosed with an LCL (Lateral Collateral Ligament) tear. However, they were not exactly sure and said that I would have to consult an orthopedist. Throughout that night, I continued feeling pain, but nonetheless went to school on crutches the next day.

After school the following day, I met with a physiatrist, who did an ultrasound of my knee and took X-rays. She diagnosed an ACL injury and LCL injury, and referred me to an orthopedist. The orthopedist saw me a few days later, but without the usual MRI diagnostics. The usual procedure for a suspected torn ACL is to undergo an MRI scan to determine the exact extent of the injury. Complicating my situation, however, is the fact that I wear a cochlear implant. A cochlear implant is an electromagnetic device implanted in the inner ear, used to help people with hearing loss.

Recipients of this device cannot undergo MRIs due to the powerful magnetic resonance which could compromise the implant. Consequently, my orthopedist determined the diagnosis based on the physical examination findings of hypermobility of the knee. He said that there was tearing of the ACL, LCL, and meniscus. He emphasized that the knee was unstable and that surgery was warranted. The path to recovery was going to be a long one. Even prior to the surgical procedure, I would need at least six weeks of physical therapy. The knee had to be in good shape before surgery, and I needed to be able to get around without crutches. Following the surgery and short-term recovery, I was required to undergo several additional months of physical therapy with a projected recovery time estimated minimally to be nine months.

Within two weeks of the injury, I began the pre-surgery physical therapy to strengthen my knee. The physical therapy regimen included initial stretching, massaging the muscles, riding a stationary bike for half an hour, additional stretching and icing. I was given a list of stretching exercises to do at home daily to supplement my physical therapy twice weekly visits. After about three weeks post injury, I had stopped using crutches, knowing I would have to rely on them again after surgery.

There are different ways to reconstruct an ACL tear, but for mine the surgeon used a portion of my patellar tendon, which was the approach he recommended. Monday December 6, 2010 was the date set for surgery. This was to be an outpatient surgery with the procedure to be completed in approximately two hours. I arrived early in the morning to be prepped for surgery, which included sedation under general anesthesia. When I awoke more than two hours later, I was told that the surgery was successful. I was further informed that my ACL had been completely torn, that there was also tearing in my meniscus, and that I sprained my LCL. So finally, I had a complete diagnosis.

To repair these respective injuries, the surgeon reconstructed the ACL, shaved down rough areas of the meniscus, and observed that the LCL would heal on its own. Upon shedding off the effects of the anesthesia, I did not feel any pain, since my knee was still quite numb. I could detect, however, that my leg was very swollen, so the doctors had put on tight stockings to help decrease the swelling. Around the stocking on my surgically repaired knee was a heavy brace designed to keep my knee stable. By mid-afternoon, I was released with instructions about how to care for my knee and a prescription for pain medication. I was also given a cooler pump with an attached hose through which ice cold water would flow into a cuff around my knee to reduce swelling. I went home that day once again supported by crutches. My mobility was limited, and in particular, negotiating stairs was very difficult, so I remained on the lower level of my home, spending the next two days and nights on the couch.

On the day following surgery, the numbness in my knee started to subside. I began to feel some pain, for which I took oxycodone. When I needed to get up (with the use of crutches), I found even small movements very painful. The combination of swelling, the tightness of the stockings, the heavy brace, and my weakness made it feel like my leg was weighted down by a block of cement.

The pain, already reduced by the pain medication, was bad when I needed to move around, and intermittent when my knee was stationary. There were times when the pain was intense, and there were other times when it was tolerable. By day three, I began using a continuous passive motion (CPM) machine, which I was instructed to use for a total of twelve hours a day for duration of about a week. The machine is designed to gradually condition the knee to resume normal bending and flexing motion. The leg rests on a cushion that is on top of a device that moves the knee up and down repeatedly at a selected angle. I initially set the machine so that my knee was only slightly bent, and over the course of the week, I increased the bend of the angle. I successfully used the machine for approximately one week. Though nowhere near fully recovered, I felt ready to return to classes after missing six school days. When I got back to school on the following Tuesday, I did so with the support of crutches. I continued using both crutches for the next three weeks, and then relied on a single crutch for an additional week, but still needed to walk slowly and cautiously.

With the passing of time and consistent physical therapy I began to regain my strength. The post-surgery physical therapy was similar to the pre-surgery PT. Starting again, from the beginning, I was given exercises to do at home, which included stretching and leg lifts. At physical therapy, I did these as well as the stationary bike. As I regained strength through home exercises and through formal physical therapy sessions, I added weights for the leg lifting

174

exercises, according to what I felt my leg could endure, and noticed that my ability to flex was improving. I remember these exercises being very tiring and there were times I felt the need to reduce the intensity. One odd suggestion that I found very helpful was to ice my knee with bags of frozen vegetables, which conforms to the shape of a knee.

Icing the knee after exercises really helped, however, walking was difficult immediately following physical therapy. In general, it took time to get my leg back into a rhythm. This was especially noticeable upon waking up in the morning. During this phase of the first few months after surgery, I would continue to feel occasional pain. This discomfort, however, was a vast improvement compared with the pain I felt in the early weeks after surgery.

In the last phase of physical therapy (approximately the fourth month), I moved from the bike to the treadmill as I was now able to run. Within a few weeks, I progressed to balancing exercises and the use of other more intense machines. I finished my physical therapy at the end of the school year in 2011, but I still had to continue running every two to three days, which I did in the summer. When I didn't stick to the schedule or pushed off exercising for an additional day or two, I would feel occasional tinges of pain. When I felt this pain, I knew it was time to exercise, and doing so made a noticeable difference. At this point, in the beginning of the summer, I was fitted with a post-surgery brace, which I was instructed to wear when doing any form of intense activity.

Six months after surgery, I was running about once a week. The protocol also included running drills that involved quick lateral movements for returning to sports. I never really got to the point where I increased the intensity of my workouts beyond running because I took a pre-college gap year to study abroad and didn't have the time and physical space to do step up the rehab. With high school behind me, however, I knew I wouldn't be returning to team sports anytime soon. I did participate in intense hiking during my year abroad, and on these occasions I wore my brace. I really learned the benefits of wearing the brace, definitely feeling how extensively the brace helped and supported my knee. On shorter and less intense hikes, I didn't wear the brace, and on these occasions, my knee would feel tired. I knew that if I had continued walking without the brace, it would have been hard to complete the hike. After both the short and long hikes, my knee would feel tired and I was in some pain. With stretching and exercising, the pain subsided.

By the end of my year abroad, approximately one and a half years after surgery, I could feel no difference between my knees. I got to the point where I had to think for a second about which knee had been injured and surgically repaired. Now it has been more than two years after my surgery. I continue to exercise and move around actively in my current college life.

Luiz, 50-year-old Male

I was 50 and playing soccer. As I was turning my body to the right, I was hit from behind in the left knee. My leg was planted so my knee twisted. I had to be helped up and could not continue playing. There was pain right away, followed by swelling overnight. I could not walk properly the next day, and it was painful to put weight on the injured leg.

I looked for a sports medicine doctor the next day, who ordered an ultrasound, followed by an MRI. The diagnosis was a partial ACL tear. The doctor recommended physical therapy to recover strength and flexibility, and surgery afterwards. The doctor recommended no soccer before the surgery because of the risk of my knee buckling and causing damage to other parts of my knee.

The doctor added that I would not need surgery if I was prepared to quit soccer or other sports requiring pivoting movements of the knee, like volleyball, basketball, tennis, squash, skiing, etc. In the meantime, I should only do straight running, hiking, and biking. I felt very well after six months of physical therapy.

As I only had a partial tear of the ACL, I looked for a second opinion. I was told to strengthen my leg muscles, try to play soccer again and practice skiing. As I was able to play and ski, I decided to heed the second doctor's opinion and decided not to have surgery.

Two years later, while playing soccer again, my knee gave out and I badly damaged my medial meniscus. The knee was locked for three months; and I could not straighten my leg. I concluded that there was no other choice but surgery.

The doctor recommended a hamstring graft because that was his expertise. They also recommended a nerve block pre-surgery but I declined, taking just ordinary anesthesia that put me to sleep for the four hours during the surgery. They replaced my ACL and also cut out the damaged part of meniscus.

The pain was really bad for the first week after the surgery, and I stayed at home, icing, and walking with crutches. I used prescription pain killers for a week but it caused constipation, so I switched to over-the-counter painkillers. I gave up the crutches after two weeks, and after two months I was able to walk without pain.

I did physical therapy for eight months, two or three times a week. The injured knee (left) is much improved but it is not the same as my good knee. My left leg is weaker, and that makes me more prone to injuries like pulled muscles.

Unless you are prepared to give up your favorite sports, undergo surgery as soon as possible. The ACL is very important to normal stability and you won't be able to practice sports without it. Schedule your surgery before damaging other parts of your knee, like the meniscus.

Finally, you should realize that no matter how successful the surgery and recovery is, your damaged knee will never be the same. The doctors will say it will be same but their knees were not injured. Still, surgery is definitely worth it. I am now 53 and feeling great.

Tammy, 55-year-old Female

On a Friday in February 2009, just before my 55th birthday, I was playing a social game of tennis. Turning to hit a backhand, my knee turned but my foot didn't, and I fell down. I did not hear the "pop" that everyone says you hear, however, there was excruciating pain. I immediately iced the knee so there was little swelling. For the next two days, I was unable to put my full weight on that leg without turning my foot sideways to redistribute the pressure.

I went to Walk-In clinic that day when I got home and was told that it didn't look like a torn ACL. A week later, I made an appointment with a sports orthopedic practice, who ordered an MRI that came back inconclusive.

Because of my age I elected to try to rehab the knee with physical therapy. I continued the rehab for three months until May of the same year, but I found that the PT was not helping. I couldn't move from side to side without terrible pain, so I finally opted for surgery and ACL replacement.

I had the surgery on May 21, 2009, as out-patient at Mt. Auburn Hospital: in at 9:15 AM and out by 1:30 PM. The torn ligament was replaced with a cadaver ligament. I went home to my CPM (continuous passive motion) machine which I dutifully used as instructed – about four hours a day. I used pain meds for one day, but they made me feel woozy, so I gave them up. The pain was not horrible. I was able to walk without crutches after two days, and subsequently used the brace they put on my leg after the operation. I had to drive an automatic for two weeks after the operation because I couldn't depress my clutch.

With Memorial Day on May 25th, I couldn't schedule my post-op appointment with the surgeon until June 2, 2009. Because of this, I didn't start PT until June 8th. I believe that due to this delayed start of my rehab program, I was never able to hyperextend my leg. I come extremely close, but I just can't do it. Had I started PT earlier, I might have made a complete recovery. This has not impeded my use of my knee/leg, but it makes me a bit upset. I did PT for about 9 months.

I also think that I was not given clear instructions on how to use the brace – what setting to use, not to put my leg on pillow no matter how much it hurt, etc. I think this also impeded my ability to hyperextend my leg and have a complete recovery. It seems crucial to get the leg to hyperextend as soon as possible after surgery – if possible still while using the CPM machine.

I can do everything I need to do, including playing tennis, basketball, rowing, etc. At this point I feel little difference between Larry (my name for my new ligament) and my good knee. Sometimes when the weather changes my bad knee will have a twinge or ache, but nothing that causes me to reduce my activity.

All in all, my ACL replacement operation and recovery went very smoothly.

Ben, 22-year-old male

I blew out my left ACL playing Ultimate Frisbee in Albany, NY in the spring of 1998, when I was 22 years old. It was a contact injury. I jumped to grab a disc, it bounced off of my hands (I really should have had it), and before I could turn to go for it an opposing player crashed into my left leg. It hurt like all heck, but I was able to slowly walk off of the field before deciding to go to the hospital.

I didn't find out that the ACL was torn until the fall of 1999. Because I was in Massachusetts and my parent's insurance was based in NJ, all they approved was a single visit to a nurse practitioner when the injury occurred. No MRI, X-ray, or anything. Since I was walking pretty well by then, they diagnosed me with a dislocated kneecap and sent me on my way. Soon after I moved to Arizona and got my own health insurance. I found myself falling down when I was running - even straight-line running – so I got a second opinion with the new health insurance. They examined me and ordered an MRI, which confirmed a torn ACL. I was scheduled for surgery in January 2000, about three months after the diagnosis and more than 18 months after the original injury. I remember being happy that it was after Y2K! The choice for surgery was a no-brainer for me. I did not want to spend years worrying about my knee giving out on me.

I think the graft was from my patellar tendon but I am sure it was not a donor tendon. My doctor never gave me a choice about this - he just stated that this was what was going to be done.

The pain wasn't terrible, but I basically was in bed for about a week after the surgery – using Percocet when necessary, and using a range of motion machine to stretch my knee out. After two weeks, I was back at work, able to drive (b/c it was the left knee), and using crutches. After a month, I was off the crutches and able to walk small distances using a brace. At three months, I continued to use a brace for long distances, but not for short distances. After six month, I started to play Ultimate again... but very slow and deliberate in all movements. After a year, I had no practical restrictions, but still didn't feel 100%. Two years after surgery, I pretty much was back to normal.

I went to PT regularly for all of my appointments over a period of approximately four months, but I did not do all the at home exercises as much as I should have. The PT really helped me extend to full range of motion and also built up some strength. Although my knee gave out a number of times out between the initial injury and surgery, I never experienced any instability after surgery.

It's been 13 years since the surgery. The surface nerves never fully regained their sense, so even today if I touch my left knee, it feels a bit desensitized. Once in a while the knee just feels "off" for a day or two - not enough to stop any activities, but just enough so that I know something had been done years ago. Sometimes I wear a knee sleeve when playing basketball, but I really don't need.

My advice is that if you plan on staying active, get the surgery done. Full recovery (100%) probably takes 18-24 months, but you can do most activities (at least lightly) within 6-9 months.

Hannah, 15-year-old Female

The summer before I entered my sophomore year of high school, when I was 15 years old, I tore my ACL at soccer camp. In late August 2008, the day began like any other with the team doing a warm up along with stretching. About halfway through the practice, we started an exercise that involved a pair of players sprinting towards the far goal, racing each other to the ball. The player who got to the ball first tried to shoot the ball at the net to score a goal. When it came to my turn, I had no problem getting to the ball and making a goal. After waiting in line, it was my turn again. My opponent and I were told to go and I sprinted as hard as I could to the ball.

I was first to the ball, and planted my right foot next to ball preparing to kick with my left. I felt a weird sensation in my planted leg, but I still managed to kick with my left leg. The ball didn't go as far as I planned, so I had to take a few steps and then kick the ball again. When I took those first couple of steps something didn't seem right, and I felt a little off balance. I ignored the fact that something might be wrong with my right leg, and instead jogged with a slight limp back to where the team was and once again waited for my turn. I kept bending and flexing my right leg because once again things just didn't feel normal. After a little while I sat on the ground and tried to stretch out my leg because I thought maybe my muscles were just stiff.

Once again, I took my turn in the game we were playing, but this time as I ran towards the ball, I felt a little bit of pain in my knee, and I felt somewhat unstable. I managed to keep going, but I had to limp my way back to where the team was, and at that point I could tell there was something wrong with my leg, so I took a break and sat down. I thought that it was just a minor sprain or muscle ache, but my knee did look a bit swollen. I ended up sitting out of the rest of the practice and icing my knee. When it didn't feel better by the next day I realized that I needed to go to the doctor, and so I did.

When I visited the doctor, they were guessing that it was a torn ACL and an MRI confirmed it. It was officially diagnosed about two weeks after it had been torn. They recommended surgery. It was an easy decision for me to undergo surgery, because I planned on continuing to play soccer after I recovered. The doctor said that playing soccer again would be impossible without surgery.

Due to a scheduled family vacation, my parents and I decided it would be better to wait and have surgery after the trip, instead of before. It was about four months between the time of diagnosis and surgery. Since there was so much time between my diagnosis and my surgery, I ended up going to physical therapy before my surgery, trying to improve my muscle strength and flexibility beforehand. After surgery, I went to physical therapy about once or twice a week for about a month. Subsequently, I did exercises and strengthening on my own, which I think worked really well for me.

During these months before my surgery there were a number of times that my knee gave out and I would stumble; once, I even fell. When it would happen it was a bit painful, but overall it was more of a weird sensation. It felt as though my knee was slipping to one side, thereby making me lose my balance. After the surgery I never again had this problem.

For the surgery, they used some of my hamstring as the graft. I didn't want to have to use a donor graft so this was the option that allowed me to use my own body parts. The first two or three days after surgery were borderline unbearable. I could hardly move at all, and with the exception of using the restroom, I never left the couch. I was definitely in a lot of pain. I used pain killers but I tried to use them very sparingly because they mostly made me sleep all day. On about the 4th day I was feeling substantially better and could get off the couch and move around my house with very little pain.

About six or seven days after my surgery I was able to return to school, but had to use crutches to move around at all. After two to three weeks, I was able to get off the crutches, and I pushed myself very hard to be able to put weight on the leg that had surgery. Although I wasn't using crutches, it was still a little hard to walk I moved very slowly, with a bit of a limp.

After a month I was doing quite well - everyday day I was able to put more weight on that leg. There was definitely a lot of stiffness in my leg that improved very slowly over time. It was a bit painful bending my knee for quite some time, and I had to make sure I stretched and bent my leg regularly. The stretching and bending hurt a little but it was necessary to do.

After a couple of months, I felt that I was back to normal but I couldn't regain my flexibility back in that leg for well over a year. When I returned to soccer again about eight months later, I think that my abilities were still not quite back to normal, and they honestly never felt like they would ever be the same again. It may be more an issue of mind over matter, but during soccer games I always still felt a little uneasy, even though I wore a brace on my leg for extra support.

Three years after my surgery, I enrolled at UMass Amherst, I decided to join an intramural soccer club. During one of the games I was running to the ball very quickly, planted that same right foot in the ground and kicked with my left leg. As soon as my foot hit the ground I felt something go wrong, and there was immediate pain in my right knee. I had to instantly pick up my leg and sit down because I couldn't put any weight on it. Two of my teammates had to carry me off the field and back to my room because it was too painful to stand or walk. The next day, I limped to the doctor's office. They told me to rest and gave me crutches, but weren't inclined to order an MRI. I was able to walk only with crutches for the first few days, and for the next two weeks I had stiffness and some pain. I could tell that something wasn't right, so about two weeks later I went home and got an MRI from my doctor. The MRI showed that I had torn my meniscus, and my doctor scheduled surgery on that same right knee for a date about three weeks after the injury.

I came home from school a day before the scheduled surgery, had the surgery the following day, and returned that same day back to school. This surgery was not as bad as having my ACL repaired, and there was much less pain. I was on my own at school, and had to take care of myself with no assistance, so I found that using the painkillers was very helpful. I mostly slept through the first day or two after the surgery, but I was much more comfortable than I was after the ACL surgery. I used crutches for only a couple of days, and after about a week I was able to go off them completely. I recovered much more quickly from this surgery, but my flexibility went back to being terrible, and there was much stiffness present in my knee.

I did all of my own muscle strengthening and stretching and didn't go to physical therapy at all this time. I recovered well, but once again it has taken a long time for things to feel normal, and now, five years from my first surgery and two years since the second one, I think my knee is finally feeling almost completely normal. There are times when the weather makes it feel stiff, and I don't feel like I have complete or full control of the muscle behind my thigh, but overall my knee feels great. It is definitely hard to tell the difference between the two. The one that had surgery does get stiff on occasion and can sometimes "click" when I exercise, but my other knee does that as well, just not as often. My back-thigh muscle on the leg that had surgery seems to have some long-term strength and control issues that I have been working on, but only time will tell if that problem will eventually disappear.

In retrospect, my advice would be to try to do some physical therapy *before* you have surgery. Getting ahead on the muscle strengthening played a big role in my quick recovery. If you are uncomfortable and are having pain, don't be afraid to use the painkillers; you will realize that after two or three days you may not even need them at all. Try stretching as much as possible, my flexibility deteriorated so quickly, and the only way I got it back way by stretching daily.

Calvin, 37-year-old Male

Fifteen years ago, I tore my ACL while playing ultimate Frisbee when I was 37 years ago. The injury occurred when I made a cut that I had executed many times in the past without any consequences. Before the game, I had stupidly been icing my hamstring due to a contusion, and I failed to warm up the hamstring properly before playing, so I suspect that my hamstring did not engage as it should have when I tried to cut, leaving my knee vulnerable. As I cut, my knee buckled, and it was clear that something was wrong, but there was no pain and little swelling, so I kept playing. I later tried to land on my bad knee while coming down from a jump, and it buckled a bit again.

When I returned home after the tournament, my doctor did the Lachman test and immediately told me that I'd torn my ACL. A subsequent MRI confirmed the tear. I am an active and wanted to be back to form as soon as possible, so I did not delay treatment. I was diagnosed on July 14, 2000, and surgery was scheduled for August 2, 2000. We decided on a patellar tendon autograph replacement.

My recovery was long but smooth. I took pain medication for the first day or two, but after that I didn't use anything. For the first week after surgery, my wife drove me around, but by August 9th I was driving myself to work. I flew for business a few weeks later, and a couple of days after that, I was off of my crutches and I was ready for serious rehab.

I worked extremely diligently, so my rehab went very well. By mid-September, I started a tiny amount of jogging on a treadmill, and by December, I played ultimate again. My last visit with my physical therapist was on January 8, 2001, about 5 months after my surgery. I played my first tournament a month later. My knee has never buckled again since the surgery.

After my surgery (at age 37), I was told that my cartilage looked great, "like the knees of a 21-year-old." By 2006, probably because of my weights and plyometric exercises, I started to have swelling in my reconstructed knee. I ended up having a Baker's cyst, which resulted in significant deterioration of my articular cartilage. My physician said that my knee now looked like the knee of a 65-year-old (I was 43).

Apparently, my knee had not been aligned properly during surgery, and all the weights and plyometric exercises (and ultimate Frisbee) had cut away a lot of my cartilage. Since that time, I have been unable to strengthen my injured leg on par with the good leg. I can feel the loss of cartilage, but with various treatments and supplements, I'm still running and playing ultimate.

My doctor claims that the misalignment of my kneecap was not caused by the autograft, but I have suspicion that it may be easier to align the knee more accurately with an allograft. If this is true, then I would have chosen that option, as the most important thing for me is long term outcome.

Lesley, 44-year-old Female

I am a forty-four-year-old woman, who tore her ACL playing soccer. Yes, playing soccer. Like many who have had this injury, I knew precisely when it occurred. Incidentally, my husband and I share the same orthopedic surgeon, but more about that later in this tale.

I have always been athletic and extremely competitive. Even as a baby, my mom often commented on how strong I was. Growing up in a very noncompetitive environment, it became very obvious to everyone how much I enjoyed playing games and winning. What to do with this energy? Like every mom in the neighborhood, she sent me (and my sister) out to play with all the other kids. It was always some kind of game ranging from kickball, "kick the can", tag football, basketball, etc. It was just great. There was unspoken respect for me and my competitive edge, especially from the boys who often dictated play. Nobody ever made me feel different because I was a girl. I can't recall if I was ever picked first, but I do know that I was never picked last on any team.

When I was in 3rd grade, my mom signed me up to play in our town's softball league, called "The Lassie League." I was placed on the team, and loved every aspect of playing an organized sport. I was a natural, and known for my hitting. The whole experience fed even more into my competitiveness, as well as my ego.

When I reached junior high, about ten years after title IX, girls' soccer was starting to take hold. I never played soccer before, but because it was the only sport offered in the fall, I immediately signed up for it. It was fun, competitive and, once again, I was playing on a team. Another thing I liked about soccer was that it allowed for individuality by creating your own "one-on-one" moves. However, it did require a lot a running and as it turned out, I wasn't in that great shape. So once again, those competitive juices started flowing, and I spent the following two summers training to play the sport better.

Coming into pre-season practices of my freshmen year, I was running a 6-minute mile, and was a very fast sprinter. I made the varsity team, along with eight other freshmen. We were a very talented group, dominating our division, and going undefeated until tournament time. The ultimate experience was winning the Western Massachusetts sectional during my senior year and making it to the state final. Unfortunately, we lost the state final 1 – 0, ending our undefeated season. It was a painful loss, but I wouldn't trade it for the world. It was all about the process and it only made the joy of winning even better.

By the time I graduated from high school, I played all four years on the varsity soccer team, scoring 56 goals and making 48 assists. I also played five seasons on the varsity softball team. Since we were a small school district, junior high students were eligible to play at the high school level. In addition, I also played three full seasons on the varsity basketball team, averaging 12 points a game, but not loving the sport as much as I loved both soccer and softball.

I was coming to the conclusion of what I thought was my athletic career. I had always been an excellent student and was prepared to make the transition to college. A free tuition ride at UMass-Amherst was available, since my dad was a professor there, but I realized that I wasn't "big enough" to play Division I sports. However, my coach, who happened to be my guidance counselor, suggested I consider Division III schools. As it turned out, a few were looking at me to play soccer and softball. In the end, I decided on one of these schools, and was able to put together a decent financial aid package. Best of all, I was able to play my two favorite sports for another four years.

After college, I enrolled in graduate school, became a mathematics teacher, married, had two children, and I stopped playing sports, or so I thought. It is funny how you end up making friends through your children. As it turned out, there were a few women (other moms) playing soccer who were looking for more players, so I became really interested, even though I hadn't played in over 10 years.

It was great to reconnect to something that I thought I would never be able to do again. This was especially satisfying because I was in a funk, bogged down by the monotony and routine of everyday life. Playing again revitalized my individuality, and allowed me to experience that rush of adrenalin that only comes with playing sports.

So there I was at my usual Tuesday night indoor soccer match, January 3rd, 2012, when I tore my knee. I didn't collide with anyone, nor fall down. All I did was raise my leg to bring the ball down, when I heard a slight "pop," and down I went. There was no pain, no swelling, but definitely not right. I was scared. I had never been seriously injured before. My husband, however, already had had two ACL surgeries, 20 years apart, one on each knee, with the most recent surgery in 2010. So I knew, more or less, what to expect.

Finding an orthopedic doctor was no issue, since we had already been through it with my husband's knee. A friend of ours also had his knee repaired, and highly recommended this same surgeon. The MRI confirmed what the surgeon had already suspected. I had a torn ACL, along with medial and lateral meniscus tears.

My doctor recommended that I see a physical therapist to assess when I would be ready for surgery, if I elected to go that route. Surprisingly, this surgery was to be totally my decision. You can live with a torn ACL, but it depends on how active you want to be. There was no question in my mind that I was going to have the surgery.

The surgeon was very clear on which physical therapist he wanted me to see and fortunately, the therapist was close to home. After the PT saw me, he wasn't surprised that I tore my ACL. Apparently, between my hips, quads, and hamstrings, everything was very tight, which puts additional strain and torque on the knees. So, after seeing him for eight pre-surgery visits, I was ready for the operation on February 14, 2012 – Happy Valentine's Day to me! Between the surgery and subsequent physical therapy sessions, recovery would be about nine months, with the "goal" for me to play soccer again.

It has been a long recovery process. You have to commit to a rigorous rehabilitation process. It is a curious injury, because you would think that the more you rest the better the knee would feel, but I have found just the opposite; the more I train and stretch the better it feels.

Would have I preferred not to have surgery? Of course! But, I'm thankful every day that the health insurance covered most of the expenses. Moreover, because of the amazing advancements in this kind of surgery, I am left me with only a one-inch scar, just below my kneecap. The very fact that I was actually able to have my knee repaired at all has allowed me to play sports once again and for that, I am thankful.

Peter, 31-year-old Male

My physical therapist Peter, a fit 31-year-old male soccer player, partially tore his ACL when he was 25. The injury swelled immediately and he was unable to play for a number of weeks. When he tried to play again, he felt looseness in the knee and was unable to push hard on it, but experienced no instability. An examination confirmed laxity in the injured knee, but a firm endpoint indicated that the ACL was intact but partially torn.

An MRI was inconclusive, but surgery was scheduled quickly so that the recovery would not interfere too much with his soon to start physical therapy training. After careful thought and a conversation with the surgeon, Peter decided to cancel the surgery. The surgeon's recommendation was that he should get back to soccer, and see what happens. If the tear was really only a partial tear, then it would be better for him to tear the ligament all the way through himself playing soccer rather than to have the surgeon cut it for him.

Playing briefly with a sports brace but not liking its feel, he soon returned to soccer without the brace and quickly resumed his normal schedule playing in a number of leagues simultaneously. Swelling subsided and the leg naturally grew strong again. This turned out well, because the knee subsequently never showed any signs of instability, and the ACL still hasn't torn any further. He is playing soccer as good as ever six years later. To this day, he can feel a difference in his two knees, but it has no effect on his athleticism. He competes with players ten years his junior. His strong soccer legs may be enough to stabilize his partially torn ACL indefinitely.

Andrea, 32-year-old Female

I injured my knee in my early 30's in three separate incidents that at the time did not seem related. The first injury occurred on a hiking trip with a friend in West Virginia, where we spent all day walking up and then back down a mountain. It was a strenuous hike and our legs felt like jello by the time we got back down. We had to walk about a half-mile or so on a flat, crushed rock path to get back to our car, and at some point, I tripped and fell. I remained on the ground for a few minutes, feeling the fall in my knee, and I limped back to the car once I was able to get up. I didn't notice any swelling or anything. The irony of walking up and down a mountain and then tripping on the way back to the car was not lost on me.

My second knee injury happened in the driveway. Our driveway sat on a small hill with a carport on top. One day, I pulled in, opened the car door, and for whatever reason, the car started rolling back down the hill. Seeing the open door moving toward the support post for the carport, I stuck my left leg out the car door - as if I was going to be able to stop the rolling car that way! About a second later I realized I could pull the emergency brake, but my knee had already suffered the brunt of my panic.

The final incident took place in NY at a rehearsal for a skit at a conference. My character was supposed to jump out and scare another. I jumped, and on the landing, I felt something in my knee snap. My knee swelled up and that was it. But before I was really down for the count, adrenaline and a strong drink got me through the performance (without the jump). I knew nothing was broken or even sprained; but the knee was huge and painful, with intense swelling. I could barely walk, so my friends found a wheelchair at the hotel. The next day I was on a bus back to DC and I made an appointment with a great orthopedist the following day.

What I do remember clearly was a diagnostic test where the doctor pulled my shin away from my thigh just as one might pull out a dresser drawer. That sort of freaked me out, but for my doctor, it was definitive in terms of diagnosing my torn ACL. I don't remember any MRI, but there must have been one because I recall the doctor wanting to order some tests to rule out other damage. The other part of this drama was that I was supposed to fly to Israel on two days later. The doctor drained my knee to reduce the swelling, and told me to wear a brace just to keep things stable. He gave me the okay to travel and told me come back three weeks later and talk about next steps.

When I got back from Israel, my doctor told me that I could have surgery, or leave it all alone. He explained that if I left it alone, I would probably be fine, *but* my knee would be less stable and I would be more likely to get arthritis in my knee later in life. My tendency to injure my knee made me fearful of future damage, and I did not like the uncertainty of going through life with a bum knee, so I chose surgery.

The big surgery question for me was repair or replacement. I chose replacement and got a cadaver ACL. I was told that replacement would be stronger than repair, and since I chose surgery for the stability, that made sense to me. I did have an option of using a graft from my own body. My doctor said that there was no intrinsic benefit to that option over the others and in my opinion, it would be one more thing my body had to heal, so I went with the cadaver replacement. I was also told that the surgery could result in minor nerve damage that would cause numbness that might or might not go away with time. In the end, I still feel a little numbness there, but it's gone down over the years and is only noticeable if I'm looking for it.

The time between diagnosis and surgery was about three months. My doctor didn't feel it was something that needed to be done as an urgent matter, and I was walking around just fine, so I waited until it was convenient for me.

After the surgery, I was on painkillers for a few days. I'm not a fan of them in general; I took them mainly at night, so I could sleep more easily.

They gave me two pieces of equipment to take home from the hospital with me. One was a cooler that was filled with ice and cold water, with a tube running to a cuff I wore around my knee. I used this for 20 minutes every two hours, and my knee was freezing - I hated that. The other thing I got from the hospital was a machine that bent and straightened my knee for about 20 minutes every two hours or so, including the middle of the night. I also hated that. My poor husband Ronnie was managing all of this for me - getting the ice and helping me get my knee in and out of the torture devices.

The worst time after surgery was when I first tried to go to the bathroom. We had a relatively small bathroom. The toilet was up against the tub, and I didn't have anywhere to put my braced (straight) leg! It was scary, strange, embarrassing, and panic-inducing. Our other bathroom was more comfortable but farther away from the bedroom where I spent most of my time the first few days. At my first follow-up appointment, I told the surgeon that he needed to warn people before the surgery that managing basic bodily functions, even ones not necessarily related to your knee, is going to be a challenge.

I stayed home from work the first week and got rides for the week or so after that. I think I had crutches for two weeks, but I hated them, and used them as little as possible. Our car was stick shift, and so I couldn't drive until I got rid of the brace and had decent mobility in my leg - I think that was after three or four weeks.

I started PT at an outside facility during week two. I went two or three days a week for the first few weeks and they were amazing. I went from thinking I would never ride a bike again to being confident that I could do whatever I wanted. I think I had six or eight weeks of rehab, and I loved seeing how much I had improved from the previous week with regard to strength, flexibility, and endurance.

By the end of two months or so, I felt really good. Not quite ready to run a marathon, but my knee had full range of motion and my muscles were getting stronger. I can't remember when I stopped thinking about my knee and protecting it and not pushing myself, but it happened faster for me than it did for those around me.

I've never had my knee give out since the surgery and these days, when I mention to people that I had ACL surgery, I have to look at my knees to remember which one. There's only a small 1" scar and I almost never think about it. And, there's a little numb patch just under my knee on that leg, but again, that's not an issue.

My advice to someone with a torn ACL: if you have the insurance, get the surgery and do the rehab. And don't do the surgery if you're not committed to the rehab. Here is another helpful tip: if you can get someone to help out for the first two weeks after surgery, then go for it. I had a friend come to town after surgery to help take care of Ronnie and me; she went shopping and cooked up a storm for us. My last piece of advice - figure out the bathroom thing!

There was some national news about a year after my surgery that cadaver parts used for surgeries were possibly infected with HIV and/or Hepatitis (I can't remember which). I didn't hear from my doctor that I was at risk and I made the decision to assume that everything was fine with my cadaver ACL. I am 47 today and the replacement ACL is holding up fine.

Ralph, 15-year-old Male

Fifteen-year-old Ralph tore his ACL playing basketball and had subsequent episodes of instability. He had ACL reconstruction using an allograft. Unfortunately, the graft got infected, and despite attempts using antibiotics to kill the infection, the graft needed to be removed. He waited a few months until he was healed, and repeated the procedure with another allograft. The second procedure was done at a different hospital, but unfortunately and surprisingly, the new graft also became infected and had to be removed. It is very rare for an allograft to fail this way, but the infections were different strains and the allografts were from different tissue banks, so it seems like a case of sheer bad luck - lightning striking twice.

The infections damaged the menisci and some surrounding bone. A bone graft was done to repair the missing bone, the damaged menisci were removed, and an ACL replacement using a hamstring autograft was performed. Later, the menisci were replaced with cadavers' menisci in a procedure called meniscal allograft transplantation.

Two years after surgery, Ralph had no pain and can function normally. However, the damage done to his knee during the two failed surgeries made it inadvisable for him to participate in sports. Hard twisting sports will eventually bring on arthritis and the more he does, the faster the pain will accelerate.

Elly, 19-year-old Female

Elly was playing softball. The bases were loaded and the count was full. She was thinking to herself - I hope the ball is hit to me. Like most good athletes, she welcomed the pressure. Amazingly, a line drive was hit in the gap near her position in the outfield, and she dashed over to make the catch. Just as she was closing her glove, her foot snagged and she tripped, allowing the ball to sail over her head. She heard a distinct pop and she fell on the floor with her leg in a bent position. Her friends and family could not figure out how she missed the catch – something she never does – and why she was lying on the floor looking as though she was laughing. Another player, backing her up, picked up the ball and made a play, and then ran over to check on Elly. By this time her friends and family, concerned about her, were also out on the field. She was not laughing – she was crying and couldn't move her leg, which was extremely painful.

Elly had a hamstring replacement. Her early recovery was difficult, but she was running after three months, and went on an overseas program after six months. Although she felt strong and was progressing, her knee still swelled badly after workouts. Eventually, she was examined and it was determined that the replacement ACL was lax and ineffective.

She scheduled a second surgery with a patellar replacement. She had a poster-child recovery the second time.

Joe, 35-year-old Male

Joe tore his left ACL when he was 18 and decided not to have surgery. For a few years he did well, but after a while he experienced progressive pain and instability. The pain eventually affected his work, recreation, and day to day life. At age 35, he decided to get treatment. At this time, his good knee measured a normal 4 mm of tibial shift, but the bad knee was very loose, measuring 13 mm. An MRI confirmed no ACL and a badly damaged medial meniscus. He had also developed severe arthritis and his bones were misshapen. He underwent three surgeries over a period of two to three years: one to reshape the bone, one to replace his ACL with a hamstring autograft, and one to replace the medial meniscus.

A year after his last surgery, he was able to pull his daughter around on a sled, give her a piggyback ride, and run the mandatory mile run for his job as a police officer. He had no lingering pain or instability. He was able to return to normal recreation and the high physical demands of his job as a police officer.

Chapter 7 – The History and Future of ACL Surgery

"It takes five years to learn when to operate, and twenty to learn when not to."
Anonymous surgeon

"There is no knee injury which could not be made worse by inappropriate surgical management."
Jack Hughston, Orthopedic surgeon and one of the fathers of sports medicine

The ACL is the most studied ligament in orthopedic literature. The importance of the ACL to a stable and functioning knee is well established and accepted. It is also well known that a torn ACL is not effectively repairable surgically. Nowadays, replacement of a torn ACL with human tissue is a standard surgical procedure with a very high (90%) complete success rate. And of the 10% that do not have a completely successful recovery, only 1% end up seriously worse off.[37]

Consequently, research papers today are no longer about whether or not to treat an ACL tear surgically, nor about exactly how to stabilize the injured knee. Today most papers discuss graft options, exact locations of attachment, rehabilitation, and injury prevention. There is much discussion about graft positioning and orientation, with a focus on trying to recreate the original ACL's anatomy as closely as possible.

However, even just forty years ago, an ACL tear was a devastating career-ending injury. After the initial trauma healed, an athlete found him/herself with an unstable knee that gave way or buckled unexpectedly and inconsistently. Repair was usually unsuccessful and replacement was typically only 60-70% successful partly because surgeons did not know where exactly to reattach the new graft. There is a century of history from the earliest ACL repairs to where we

---

[37] https://consultqd.clevelandclinic.org/10-year-outcomes-and-risk-factors-after-acl-reconstruction-a-multicenter-cohort-study/

find ourselves today. This chapter is a brief overview of that history. The interested reader can find more information in the referenced papers[38] [39].

The Early Years

The first clinical description of an ACL tear was by Robert Adams in 1837. The earliest attempts to heal an ACL tear occurred much later. The repair technique used direct repair; that is, the ACL was effectively reconnected by sutures. Two papers, one in 1900 by Battle and one in 1903 by Robson, described successful repairs with a two-year and an eight-year follow up, respectively. These studies were isolated and a few later studies did not replicate this success. Furthermore, a number of surgeons, such as Groves (1917), pointed out that direct repair by suturing was often impossible due to the poor condition or outright destruction of the ACL itself, and he recommended reconstruction using graft tissue. Although, not uniformly appreciated in his time, Groves was the first to replace the ACL in a manner that was in principle very similar to the way it is done today. In 1903, Lange in Munich, experimented unsuccessfully using silk to bolster the strength of the torn ACL. In 1912, also in Germany, there was a study using *xenografts* – grafts from animals. In particular, a kangaroo tail tendon was used to replace an ACL, but the results were very poor due to rejection of the graft and infections. Generally, these early studies were experimental and there was no standard surgical procedure being used for torn ACLs.

With Campbell in the 1930s and O'Donoghue in the 1950s, interest in aggressively treating ACL tears either via repair or replacement continued, but it was still not the mainstream

---

[38] An Illustrated History of Anterior Cruciate Ligament Surgery, Patrick C. McCulloch, Christian Lattermann, Arthur L. Boland, Bernard R. Bach ,Jr., **The Journal of Knee Surgery**, April 2007, Vol 20 No 2, pages 95-104, http://www.bachmd.com/Files/An%20illustrated%20history789.pdf,

[39] *Surgery for Anterior Cruciate Ligament Deficiency: A Historical Perspective*, Oliver S. Shindler, Knee Surg Sports Traumatol Arthrosc, Springer Verlag, 2011, http://ucismig.weebly.com/uploads/5/2/1/2/5212593/acl_history.pdf

to treat these injuries. Over the next 50 years, the debate regarding ACL injuries centered not so much on whether to attempt primary repair or perform reconstruction, but on whether or not to treat the injury at all. Many prominent surgeons felt that if the menisci were in good shape, and the other structures of the knee were strong, then a torn ACL could be left as is. In retrospect, they did not appreciate the crucial role that the ACL plays in preventing the tibia from moving forward relative to the femur. The importance of repair/reconstruction versus no treatment did not become apparent until the 1970s. Even then, it was still a number of years more until technique and success rates improved enough to recommend treatment to older people and to those for whom athletics was not a crucial part of their lives.

The Middle Years – Extra-Articular Reconstruction

The final blow to primary repair occurred in the 1970s. A study of West Point cadets by Feagin was presented in 1972 at the annual American Academy of Orthopedic Surgeons meeting, showing initial success with a technique called the "over-the-top" repair. However, in Feagin's five year follow up report in 1976, the cadets had developed recurrent instability and deteriorated function. Coincident to this study, surgeons began to work on techniques to reconstruct the stability of an ACL-deficient knee.

In the late 60s and early 70s, the pivot-shift deficiency (from the Pivot-Shift test) was discovered and it was felt that any technique that could avert this problem went in the right direction. In a variety of ways, ligaments were rerouted to different positions and anchored into various places in an attempt to stabilize the knee and thereby reduce the pivot-shift. This style of repair where the knee is stabilized by manipulation of various capsular structures without replacing the ACL directly is called *extra-articular* reconstruction.

201

A surgical focus on *extra-articular* reconstruction began. In the 1960s, Don Slocum and Bob Larson developed an operation called "pes plasty" that successfully rehabilitated a number of athletes. The main focus of their work was to repair the rotational instability of the knee by stabilizing the capsular structures rather than to repair the non-functioning ACL. In 1968 the great running back Gale Sayers tore his ACL after being tackled hard on a pitchout. He was treated using extra-articular techniques, and despite a tremendous effort on his part to rehabilitate his knee, his career was over. ACL tears in those days were more often than not career-ending injuries.

The Slocum/Larson technique was improved upon by Nicholas in 1973.[40] Patients were casted for six weeks after surgery in a flexed position, often resulting in long-term motion loss. A number of other surgeons, including Hughston, MacIntosh, Ellison, and Andrews, tried different and innovative extra-articular schemes, but in the long run, none of these techniques resulted in good long-term knee function.[41] In 1978, Kennedy published a landmark study [42] showing that less than half of 52 patients repaired with extra-articular techniques were able to achieve excellent outcomes with regard to stability. Warren and Marshall followed with a similar study [43] of 86 patients and similar results. Although pivot-shift was eliminated or diminished with an extra-articular reconstruction, forward tibial movement with respect to the femur was not well controlled, and many patients had unstable knees.

The various extra-articular ligament manipulations, transplants, tightening, rethreading, and repositioning eventually failed or stretched out over time. By the end of the 1970s, it had

---

[40] https://www.ncbi.nlm.nih.gov/pubmed/4800805
[41] https://www.ncbi.nlm.nih.gov/pmc/articles/PMC3560904/
[42] https://link.springer.com/content/pdf/bfm%3A978-1-4471-4270-6%2F1.pdf
[43] https://www.semanticscholar.org/paper/Injuries-of-the-anterior-cruciate-and-medial-of-the-Warren-Marshall/df89e69fffa6e66ede9f882bf3edbfba06b4aed9

become well accepted that the only effective treatment for a torn ACL was a direct *intra-articular* replacement; that is, a replacement that sits directly in the location of the original ACL.

Coinciding with the end of extra-articular techniques was the end of synthetic replacements. In particular, the failure of synthetic replacements was pronounced by Ejnar Eriksson of Stockholm, an early proponent of intra-articular patellar tendon replacements, who said of synthetic replacements in 1976, "Like shoestrings they eventually break."[44]

Modern Times – Arthroscopy and Intra-Articular Reconstruction

In the 1980s, the Lachman test and its clinical importance were described. This was supported with the knowledge that the ACL is the primary restraint of forward tibial movement relative to the femur. In response, surgeons directed their attention to a more anatomical repair of the injured ACL, and the period of intra-articular reconstruction began, that continues to this day.

The main feature of all intra-articular reconstructions is that the graft is placed more or less in the same location as the original ACL. This means somehow threading the graft through the tibial tunnel, into the notch and up into the bottom of the femur, or femoral tunnel. The "tunnels" are drilled into the bone providing a natural anchoring location for the two ends of the graft. A number of different techniques for doing this with a variety of different grafts emerged. The most popular grafts were the middle third of the patellar tendon and the hamstring tendon. In order to get the location correct, the surgery required opening up the knee, which caused more pain and slowed recovery. The introduction of arthroscopic surgical techniques allowed

[44] *Sports Injuries of the Knee Ligaments*, Ejnar Eriksson, presented at 23rd annual meeting of the American College of Sports Medicine in Anaheim, California, Med Sci Sports, 1976, 8: 133–144.

reconstructions to occur with much less soft tissue damage, less trauma, and subsequently better outcomes and recovery.

During this time period, many synthetic grafts were tried in order to avoid the secondary surgery of harvesting the graft and the resulting pain and damage therein. Among the various plastics, polypropylene, carbon fiber, and other synthetics were brand names like Polyflex, Proplast, Gore-Tex, and Dacron. None of these grafts proved successful. Every one of these grafts eventually stretched out and/or failed from excessive wear and tear. Except for use as extra support for a human tissue graft, synthetic grafts did not prove effective.

A popular idea in the 1990s was to combine a synthetic replacement with an autograft. The idea was that since a biological graft weakens and degenerates for six weeks before thriving, an artificial polypropylene *ligament augmentation device* (LAD)[45] would be inserted as backup support for the biological graft. The studies did not indicate that this was particularly effective at minimizing injury to the graft. Patients with and without the LAD had similar outcomes. This was true whether they had autograft or allograft replacements.[46]

Arthroscopy means operating through small holes using scopes threaded through the holes in order to see what you are doing. By the 1990s, arthroscopic techniques had advanced and the two popular intra-articular grafts, the patellar tendon and the hamstring, were being implemented arthroscopically through one or two small incisions, rather than via a wide open knee. This drastically minimized trauma and improved recovery times.

The focus now was on exactly where and at what angles to drill the tibial and femoral tunnels, and how to twist the graft, so as to anatomically recreate the ACL as accurately as

---

[45] *The ligament augmentation device: an historical perspective,* Kumar K., Mafulli N., Arthroscopy. May 1999;15(4), pages: 422-32, http://www.ncbi.nlm.nih.gov/pubmed/10355719
[46] *The Effect of a Ligament-Augmentation Device on Allograft Reconstructions for Chronic Ruptures of the Anterior Cruciate Ligament,* Noyes FR, Barber SD, J Bone Joint Surg Am. August 1992, 74(7): pages 960-73, http://www.ncbi.nlm.nih.gov/pubmed/1522103

possible. The goals were to avoid stretching the graft, prevent impingement of the graft by the tibia, and to not over-constrain the knee inhibiting range of motion. There was the also the issue of how to carefully anchor the ends of the graft into the two tunnels, so that the graft would not move or slip over the short or long term.

The patellar tendon and hamstring tendon presented two different problems with regard to the placement of the tunnels and the anchoring within them. The patellar tendon is harvested by removing the middle third of the tendon with two small bone fragments on the ends at the top and bottom. The top bone comes from the patella and the bottom from the tibia. This leaves the original bone to tendon connection in place and allows bone to bone anchoring with absorbable screws in the tibial and femoral tunnels.

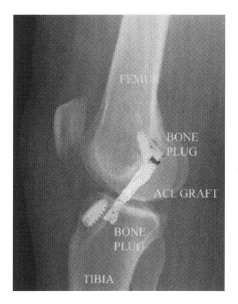

An X-ray of a Knee with Superimposed Image of a Patellar Tendon ACL Replacement

Graft[47]

[47] http://orthoinfo.aaos.org/topic.cfm?topic=A00297

In contrast, the hamstring tendon has no bones on its ends, so anchoring must be done with sutures or staples. The angle of the tunnels is more crucial with bone anchoring because a bad angle would put a great stress on the joint between the bone and tendon. On the other hand, anchoring bone to bone is stronger, heals faster, and more reliably remains in place through recovery. The choice of graft is a toss-up, and surgeons tend to specialize and become expert in one of the graft options.

By the year 2000, ACL surgical technique had evolved into a standard of arthroscopic intra-articular replacement using a patellar tendon or hamstring autograft, or an allograft. Furthermore, outcomes were excellent, with 90% of patients being fully functionally restored. However, despite all the research and techniques used to ensure the most accurate anatomical reconstruction of the ACL, studies of the knee show that replacement ACLs do not restore normal rotational kinematics. It is feared that over the long term, this altered kinematics may bring on early arthritis, but not enough time has yet passed to do careful studies.

Nonetheless, the current focus of research is to make the ACL replacement even *more* anatomically correct. One way to accomplish this is to attempt to replicate the inner structure of the ACL. It is known that the ACL contains two distinct bundles of tissue each of which tightens or loosens differently depending on whether the knee is flexed or extended. One idea is to use two grafts, one for each bundle, the so-called *double-bundle* replacement. The double-bundle replacement mimics the kinematic functionality of the ACL, so theoretically it would result in better long term outcomes. Of course, with two pieces of tissue, the surgery is more complex and errors become more common. Whether the extra work and associated risks of a double-bundle replacement is worth it is unclear. It would be preferable if one could reap the kinematic benefits of a double-bundle replacement without increased risks.

206

An alternative to a true double-bundle replacement, which attempts to reap the benefits without the risks, is to simply twist the graft 180 degrees to simulate the two bundles with one piece of tissue. This is a common clinical practice today and indeed, it was the method used by Dr. Berkson in my surgery. Future studies will indicate whether a true double-bundle replacement has measurably better outcomes than this simpler single strand simulated twist.

Another alternative nowadays is to use an allograft pre-loaded with the patient's own stem cells. The idea is to try to get the benefits of the patient's own tissue and resulting strength of the new ACL while minimizing the secondary trauma caused by hamstring or patellar grafts. Professional dancers, for example, cannot afford to lose any part of their patella tendon or their hamstrings, so this technique is perfect for a dancer's ACL replacement. The graft is placed to allow the hyperextension that dancers require. Other athletes do not need this flexibility, but without it, a dancer would not be able to perform at world-class level.

The Future

The more distant future looks toward innovative directions. One idea is to repair the ACL without cleaning out the old tissue using "growth factors", that is, tissue grown in a lab. The concept of repairing an ACL, rather than replacing it, was tried 50 years ago and resulted in complete failure. Surgical reattachment was a failure because the ACL did not regenerate effectively. However, because of advances in tissue growth and handling, these ideas are being reconsidered in the context of new technologies.

One particularly neat idea concentrates on using a synthetic "hybrid" graft as scaffolding on which the patient's own tissue can grow. When the scaffolding graft is inserted into the torn ACL, the ACL attaches to it, heals, and repairs itself. This is superficially similar to the ligament augmentation devices of the 1990s. Whereas both ideas combine biological replacements with synthetic support, the new idea allows repair rather than replacement. The new research uses a synthetic scaffolding to allow a new ACL to grow from scratch, while the old idea merely added a piece of plastic to protect dead tissue until ligamentization.

The advantage of a repair over a replacement is that a repair "preserves the complex attachment sites and innervation of these structures, thus retaining much of the biomechanical and proprioceptive function of these tissues."[48] The hybrid graft could theoretically be "built" into a more realistic ACL than any current replacement options. A second advantage of the innovative hybrid approach is that a hybrid graft avoids the need for harvesting a replacement graft and therefore allows for faster healing and less trauma. A hybrid graft has all the advantages of an allograft without any downside. Indeed, it has an upside – the new ACL is as close to the original as possible.

Another research group at Northwestern University is successfully testing a hybrid polymer ACL in animals[49]. Testing in humans is still some years off. Because outcomes from modern replacement techniques are so reliable, this new area of growth factors research will need a long time before it is considered to be a viable alternative. It would be interesting to jump ahead 50 years in the future, and look back to see what has happened to ACL surgery. Will these growth factors ideas take hold? Perhaps we will be talking about the effective, but invasive and primitive, replacement techniques of the early 21st century. We may read about how "nowadays," due to more advanced control over tissue synthesis, and via the use of a hybrid scaffolding graft and regeneration, an ACL can be effectively *repaired* rather than replaced.

---

[48] http://www.ncbi.nlm.nih.gov/entrez/eutils/elink.fcgi?dbfrom=pubmed&retmode=ref&cmd=prlinks&id=1 9064165 Current Status and Potential for Primary ACL Repair, Martha Murray, MD

[49] Northwestern Magazine, Summer 2015.

About the Author

Dr. Shai Simonson, Ph.D (b. 1958) is a professor of computer science at Stonehill College. At various times, he has taught gym, science, mathematics, and computer science to students from first grade through graduate school. Shai was the director of ADUni, http://aduni.org, which offers free computer science lectures to students all over the world, especially in developing countries. He plays go and bridge, dabbles with poker and Scrabble, loves to hike, cycle, bowl, sing, and play disc-golf. Shai grew up in New York, spent ten years in Chicago, and now makes his home in the Boston area. He spent two years (1983 and 1999) teaching and doing research in Israel. He is married with three children.

Shai tore his ACL in 2012 in a hiking accident while scrambling on some rocks. He is reminded of his strong surgically reconstructed knee with every hike, basketball scrimmage, ultimate frisbee game, and unexpected twist. It was all worth it.

His book Rediscovering Mathematics, https://web.stonehill.edu/compsci/RediscoveringMath/RM.html is available from the American Mathematical Society: https://bookstore.ams.org/clrm-39/ and Amazon: https://www.amazon.com/gp/product/0883857707/ref=dbs_a_def_rwt_hsch_vapi_taft_p1_i0

Printed in Great Britain
by Amazon

60028735R00125